MUDRAS

By

SUNDAR RUSHDIE

INTRODUCTION

Do you often feel that there is, mentally, a constipated corner somewhere in your body that's blocked mercilessly? When in distress, we all feel that block in the head!

Will power, subconscious mind power, emotional intelligence, psychic power and other varied altered sense of reality and parameters are part of a world of knowledge not known to the present progressive era. This reality cultivates a kind of energy and power to progress through enlightenment into the commonness by practicing mudra power.

The book ahead will take you through a tirade of many valuable information, benefits, effects and importance of articulating mudra power in your life. Practicing all mudras with care, knowledge and precision will help you reap all your benefits in the right time.

Good Luck!

TABLE OF CONTENTS

Book 1: 23 Mudras for Weight Loss 9

Book 2: 23 Mudras for spiritual healing 35

Book 3: 21 Mudras for Awakening Chakras 77

LEGAL NOTES

23 MUDRAS FOR WEIGHT LOSS

TABLE OF CONTENTS

Chapter 1. What are Mudras and How to utilise it for Weight Loss? 1

Chapter 2. Preparation for Mudras Training towards weight loss 3

Chapter 3. Mudras I 6

Chapter 4. Mudras II 13

Chapter 5. Mudras III 19

Chapter 6. Mudras IV 25

Chapter 7. Core Mudra: Surya Mudra 29

Chapter 8. Issues of Weight-loss through Mudra Power 32

Conclusion 34

BASICS OF MUDRAS

Mudras are part of a world that is organized and governed by the knowledge of positions, poses and meditational postures that calm, nourish and nurture the spiritual and mental energy flow and its effects in the human body. In order to start with mudras, one must have a substantial understanding of what mudras are.

What are Mudras?

Mudras are seals or forces that enhance or clear the energy flow in one's body and mind. These encompass several positions of the body along with your hand and mind when you mediate to focus and heal any part of your mental and emotional organs. These energy flow structures instills a strong and nourishing flow of energy to heal and clear out any debris or block in the body. Mudras goes well with a lifestyle that is enriched with positivity and honesty. It is within the binds and freedom of every man or woman to abide by positivity, negativity or confusion. In order to scrape the negativity and resolve the confusion, one must go through relaxed sessions of genuine meditation.

This power of mudras lays in its positive and blossoming dose of spiritual strength and for the will power to communicate non-verbally in order to invoke the impetuous power of your mind. This strength is held in the way of living and ritualizing or productively resulting on a lifestyle that is sans the sedentary aspects of robots, machines and automatons. One must research and acquire knowledge of the various acupressure and acupuncture practices as well.

How to Utilize it for Weight Loss?

Awakened, charged and trained a certain way, mudras can help a person in developing a skill or power to heal, nourish and rejuvenate any part of the physical and mental self. Utilizing this power in order to cut down on your diet is extremely helpful when you are planning to have a revised diet and lifestyle from the practice sessions.

Awakening your mental power to burn and heal your physical body requires sufficient practice and strength to continue ad blossom.

Apart from the other benefits of healing zillions of ailments, obesity can be also cured by employing the same practice. The power is enhanced when it links with the functionality of all our physical and mental organs. The weight loss secret lies within the practice of many mudras to take you to master the expert mudra or surya mudra.

There is a forthcoming chapter, focused on the supreme aspect of knowledge, theory and practice of surya mudra after training for enriching the energy flow through other mudras. These mudras take care to heal you of other illnesses, unlike other curative medicines. Many of the mudras' effects include targeting the source directly and mobilizing it.

CHAPTER 2

PREPARATION FOR MUDRAS TRAINING TOWARDS WEIGHT LOSS

At this stage of vague understanding of how mudras will focus on your weight loss aspects, I would like to introduce you to some key concepts of mudra power.

1. Metabolism: The metabolism of your body is also regularized by mudra power. The increased metabolism is an aftermath of stimulation from your activity-craving brain. The inactive and dormant glands are awakened to metabolize more and actively in your body. This helps gain more hormonal output as well as focused weight loss.

2. Mobilization: The fats in your body is exploited and energized by mudra power. Certain techniques, positions and ways of respiration affects the way your mudra gets charged-up or attains power. This results in fat that is active and enthusiastic to be burned

up. This also stimulates the respiration activity to burn off more energy from the body's powerhouse.

3. Ritualizing: All this results in a regularity or routine to affect your very life and its style of waking hours. The importance is necessary to make your mental and spiritual flow energized, awake and positive all the while as well. This has a direct connection with one's physical aspects of fulfillment, pleasure and satiation. The philosophy is the centripetal force that drives the effect to results and not merely the acts exclusively.

Preparation Physically, Mentally and Spiritually Towards Mudra Power for Weight Loss

After one is done with the right understanding of the flow of energy and its charging and energizing, he or she will have to prepare in all the domains to start the practice practically. When a person is ready from all sides, he or she gains a neat and lucid energy flow almost immediately through the mind, body and spirit channels. One should look out for disciplined and free ways of practices that allows the body to relax sans anxiety, anticipation and undue pressure.

Physical preparation

a. Prepare for a good, healthy and hygienic diet.
b. Include more grains, leaves, color and freshness of fruits to your diet.
c. Get healthy physically.
d. Exercise regularly.
e. Do breathing exercises regularly.
f. Follow a regular routine for waking up and sleeping.
g. Follow a meal plan and schedule.

h. Try consuming a non-addictive dose of nicotine, caffeine and tea.
i. Opt for spiritual clasps when losing your temper for calm control.
j. Radiate positivity through verbal and vocal thoughts.

Mental Preparation

a. Prepare for meditation.
b. Practice relaxation.
c. Practice holding your temper.
d. Practice positive self-talking.
e. Believe in the existence of your subconscious mind power.
f. Communicate with your subconscious mind.
g. Charge your subconscious mind.
h. Realize your focus.
i. Realize your potential.
j. Activate all your will power in preparation to heal yourself of all fat on your mental and physical mind and soul, respectively.

Spiritual preparation

a. One must be at peace, in the spiritual sense, with oneself.
b. Realize your positives.
c. Realize your negatives.
d. Hone your positives.
e. Start believing in yourself.
f. Start charging up your confidence.
g. Realize your potential.
h. Boost yourself.
i. Find warmth, positivity and confidence in your friends and family.
j. Celebrate your potential productively!

CHAPTER 3

MUDRAS I

Mudras are some amazing results of strong will power and mindfulness. One must acquire enriched and healthy curiosity of exploring healthy benefits and healing through mudras. The crossing, combining, fusing and bending of the energy flow and positivity through mudra practice will reap all health benefits of resolving the aches and ailments of the body.

Mudra #1

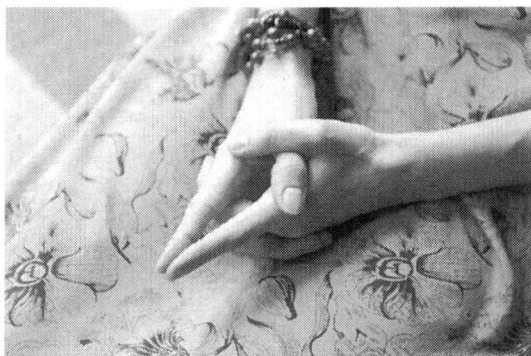

Ksepana Mudra

The mudra for letting go, ksepana mudra, is focused on pouring out energy to let go of all the negativity. The best beginning is elimination of waste as part of preparation for a healthy and proportionate physique because ksepana mudra focuses on intestinal elimination.

   a. Touch your index fingers against each other, flat.
   b. Fold the rest of the fingers against each other.
   c. Rest the remaining fingers on the back of your opposite hands.
   d. Fill in the gaps in between your thumbs by crossing them against each other.
   e. Leave a small hollow space in between the hands.
   f. Point this to the ground when seated comfortably.
   g. When lying on the ground, point it towards your feet.

Mudra #2

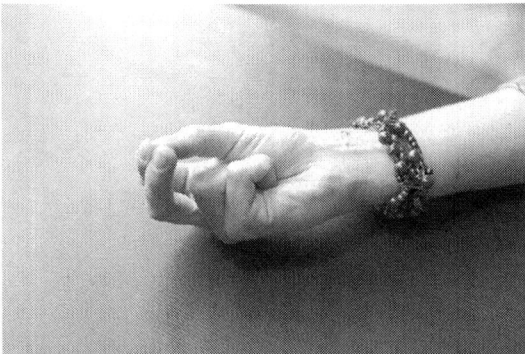

Kubera Mudra

For mental satisfaction, kubera mudra focuses on wealth. This mudra is used to ablaze the confidence, peace and serenity in choosing and doing what one is convinced of within his or her confidence. This mudra focuses on attaining a mental peace with one's possessions and being. The mudra is also used to cleanse the sinuses.

a. Place the three fingertips, index, thumb and middle finger together.
b. Fold the rest of the fingers into the center of your palm.
c. Continue and repeat with each hand.
d. Meditate and focus for a considerable time with the mudra.
e. Focus on your confidence and creativity.
f. The force gathered is of the three planets Jupiter, Mars and Saturn to revive joy, forcefulness and fixation on passing new gateways.

Mudra #3

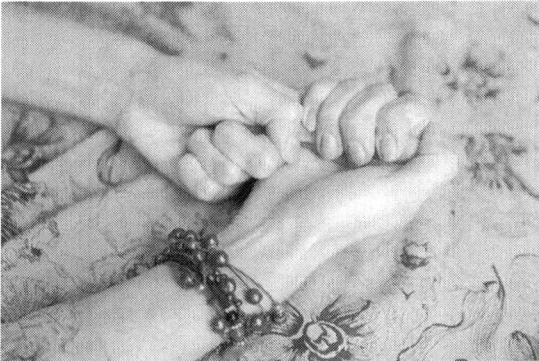

Kundalini Mudra

For awakening your sexual flow and force, kundalini mudra is used. With opposing polarity, this mudra focuses masculine as well as feminine in its power. This infuses the cosmic and spiritual soul.

a. Close both of your hands into fists.
b. Pull the index finger of your left hand into the fist of the other from below.
c. Hold your thumb pad on the fingernail of your left hand.
d. Continue this mudra for half an hour everyday and focus on your sexual awakening.
e. Keep the mudra protruded in front of your abdomen.
f. The forces revived are of the tantric yoga and focuses on awakening the sexual desire and are gratifying as well as satiates it.
g. The energy of pleasure is infused in the spiritual, mental and physical during this phase.

Mudra #4

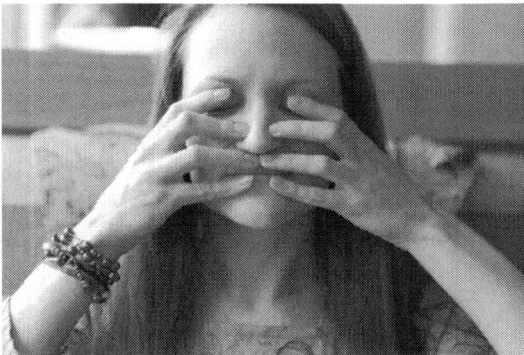

Yoni Mudra

The mudra translates to the mudra of the uterus because charging by this mudra instigates a meditative feeling of being cut off from the world as in being inside a womb or uterus. The mudra focuses on getting rid of the negativity and dishonesty of the world to enter a divine void like the womb.

a. Sit down comfortably and start meditating.
b. Breathe properly and deeply.
c. Close your ears with your thumbs.
d. Close your eyes with your index fingers.
e. Close your nostrils with your middle fingers.
f. Place your ring fingers on your lips.
g. Place your little fingers on the bottom lip close to your mouth.
h. Take your middle fingers off and exhale.
i. Inhale and close your fingers.
j. Hold the breath as a gap and feel the silence flowing in and out of you.
k. Repeat this certain number of times daily.

Mudra #5

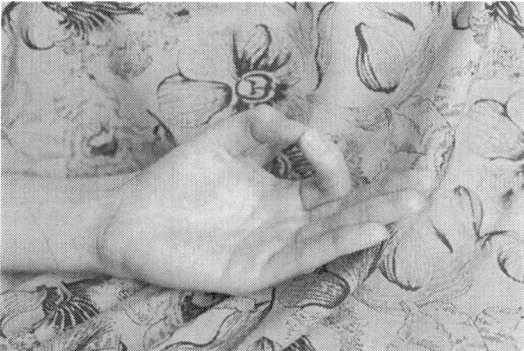

Chin Mudra

Commonly known as the jnana mudra, a gesture or seal of consciousness, knowledge is focused as well as charged with this mudra.
There are two ways of doing this mudra, both focused on the nature of consciousness through thumbs.

a. Join the thumb tip and index fingertip together.
b. Extend the rest of the fingers and point them straight.
c. Relax your hands on your thighs.
d. Continue with each hand.
e. When the fingers point towards earth, it is called chin mudra.
f. While it faces the heavens, it is called jnana mudra.
g. For the second way, apply pressure on the nails.

Mudra #6

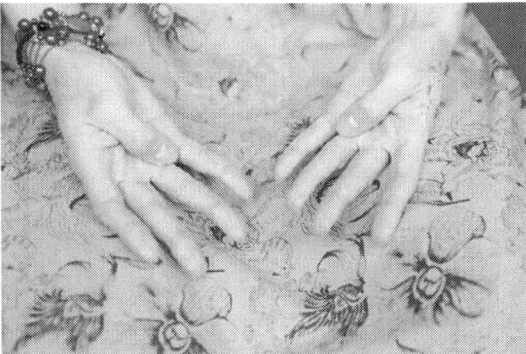

Detoxification Mudra

All of us need detoxification before we start healing our bodies. A healthy way of doing this thoroughly is through the practice of meditating on mudras. At least once a week, one should detoxify the mind and body. Make sure you rest often during your days of detoxification treatment.

a. Touch your thumb on the inner edge of the ring finger inside the palm.
b. Hold it on the last ring.
c. Continue with each hand.

11

d. Repeat this exercise for 15–20 minutes.
e. One should rest and relax many times during the same day.
f. This detoxification treatment is supposed to focus on eliminating the dirt, waste and dust from the body.
g. Relax and pamper yourself during these days.

CHAPTER 4

MUDRAS II

This chapter enfolds some of the mudras focused on a spiritual waking in order to clean and clear the debris of the mind, body and spirit. The bigger picture of this mudra power is that it can provide respiratory and other healing concoctions so that the body sheds weight and fat alongside.

Mudra # 7

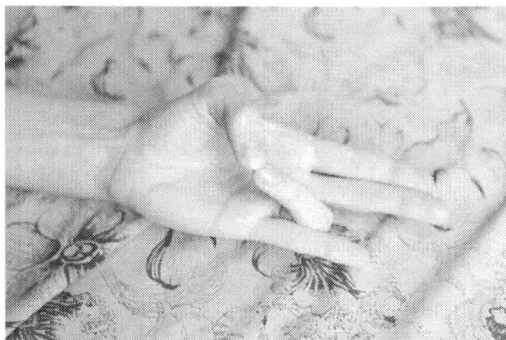

Prithvi Mudra

For uplifted belief in the self or the universe and its gravitational forces, prithvi mudra is used to strengthen all aspects of being alive for an individual.

    a. Sit comfortably or stay standing relaxed.
    b. Touch your thumb tip and ring fingertip.
    c. Point your remaining fingers straight and erect.
    d. Meditate and focus on your chakra for 20–30 minutes.

Mudra # 8

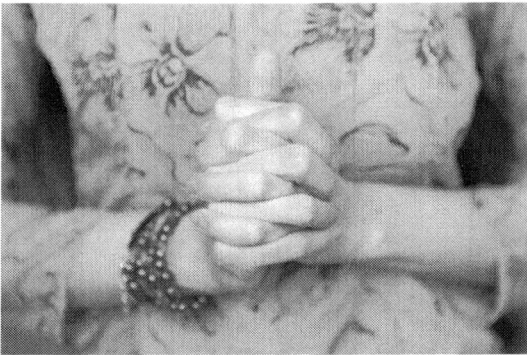

Linga Mudra

Also known as the mudra for energy and heat, this mudra is also the core mudra for stimulating the body to combat all enemies of your immune system. The mudra helps charge your body to resist all colds and fevers.

    a. Sit comfortably or stand relaxed.
    b. Intertwine your fingers around each other.
    c. Point this in front of your chest, towards the outside.
    d. Now point your thumbs straight up and erect.
    e. Hold the mudra and meditate with proper breathing exercise for 20–30 minutes daily.

f. The mudra helps focus on the loosening up of the body in order to crack everything up in your body that adds to disease or ailment.

Mudra # 9

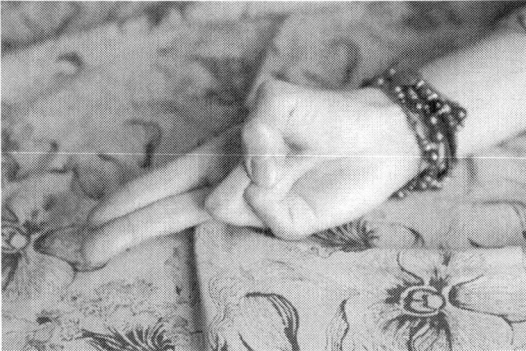

Pitta Karak

Concerned with the bodily energy of breaking down and the digestion of food, pitta karak mudra is focused on amassing heat enough for the body's energy value. This heat is used to resolve lack of enthusiasm, excitement, and low self-esteem as well as obesity in our body, mind and soul.

a. Fold your little finger and ring finger onto the ball of your thumb.
b. Now fold your thumb slowly.
c. Keep it tapped on the folded two fingers.
d. Practice the mudra for 15–20 minutes three times a day.

Mudra # 10

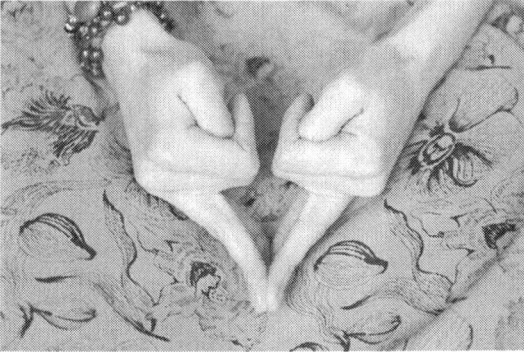

Shakthi Mudra

Honored by the goddess of energy and life, Shakthi is concerned with the strength of the mind, body and soul. The mudra is very strengthening, revitalizing and rejuvenating to the physical body and the mental spirit to heal all ailments like stress, obesity and depression.

    a. On both hands, bend your thumb toward your palm.

    b. On both hands, fold the middle finger and the index finger on the thumb.

    c. Join the fingertips of your little finger and ring finger.

    d. Meditate for some time in this position.

    e. Focus on awakening your pelvic area.

    f. Continue daily for 20–25 minutes each.

    g. The relaxation brings a new joy to be active to the pelvic area as well as the body and mind.

Mudra # 11

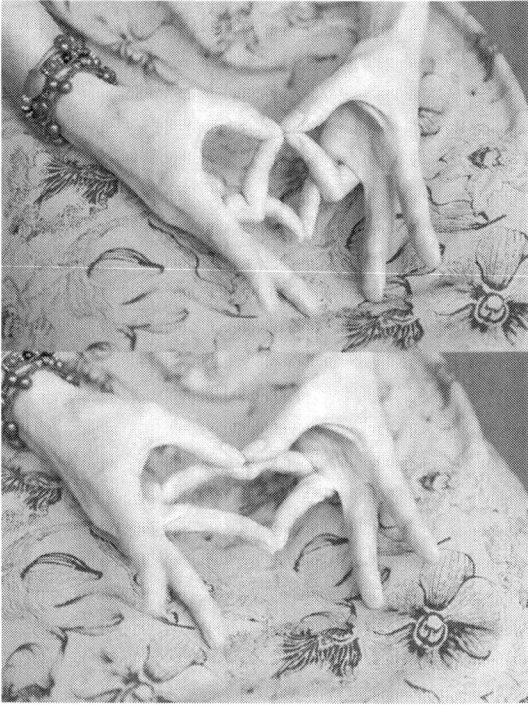

Maha Sacral Mudra

Commonly known as the large pelvis mudra, this is the posture for igniting and relieving inactive areas of the physical body and its mindset. In addition to being a good cover against menstrual aches, this mudra relieves the body of its bonds and burns excess fat as well. The mudra also provides many energy neutralizing waves to the person.

1. Touch the tips of your ring finger onto the thumb of both hands.
2. Pull together and touch the conjoined fingertips of your fingers.
3. Touch the tips of your ring finger.

4. Continue this position for 10–15 minutes.
5. Now change the position to touch your ring finger with your thumb of both hands and place the little fingers on each other.
6. Continue this for another session of 10–15 minutes.
7. Point your remaining fingers straight.

Mudra # 12

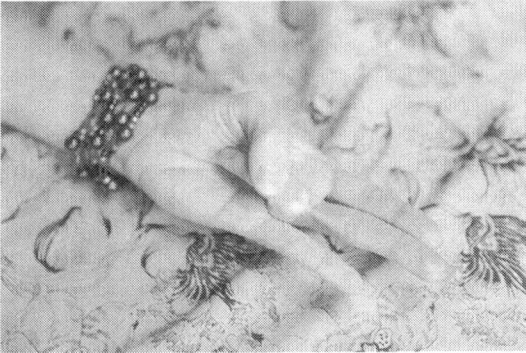

Agni Mudra

One of the prominent mudras for weight loss, agni mudra is focused on the power of fire in your body and mind. The mudra powers the digestion to speed up as well as strengthen the body.

a. Fold your ring finger.
b. Now bend your thumb and hold the ring finger underneath, gently.
c. Hold the mudra for 20–25 minutes many times daily.
d. Morning positions and breathing helps the respiratory ailment resolve on its own.
e. This mudra also helps in controlling your cholesterol levels.

CHAPTER 5

MUDRAS III

This chapter enfolds types of mudra power that is known to be the strengthening element for the earth power. Many wasted substances instill waste into the intestines, lungs and bladders throughout the journey of physical life. One must learn to live properly in order to gather the strength and power of all energy flow within and around the body as well.

Mudra # 13

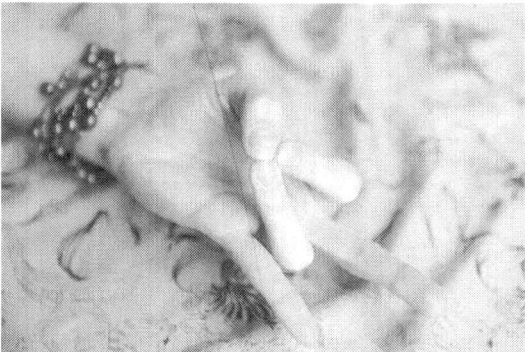

Rudra Mudra

A powerful mudra used to charge the powerful conqueror of the solar plexus, rudra mudra is used to treat many unnecessary types of sediment in the chest, pelvis or back. The mudra charges up the body to heal and resolve all blocks to clear and clean out the original physique and mental potential. Dizziness, heartaches and other fatigue-related medical ailments can be treated with this mudra.

    a. Join the tips of your ring, thumb and index finger together.
    b. Straighten out the rest of the fingers.
    c. Continue the session to focus with each hand for around 20 minutes many times daily.

Mudra # 14

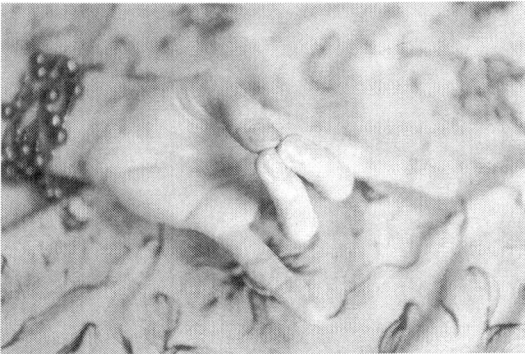

Apan Mudra

The very mudra of energy, apan mudra revives the running cogwheels of the body's energy storehouses. An absolute remedy to removing all waste and trash from your mind and body, apan mudra detoxifies the body as well. The inner balance and stability of the body and mind is maintained by this mudra and its power.

a. Join the tips of your ring, middle finger and thumb together.
b. Straighten the rest of the fingers out.
c. Relax and meditate for 15–20 minutes.
d. Repeat with each hand.
e. Do 2–3 times daily.

Mudra # 15

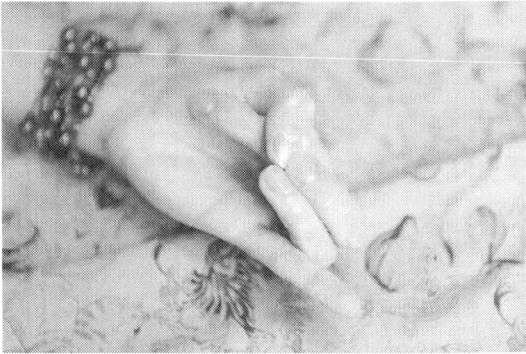

Apan Vayu Mudra

Commonly known as the mudra for saving life of one in danger, this mudra is a common first-aid technique. If the mudra is tried-out at the onset of an attack, according to the professional orator Keshav Dev, the resultant damage can be controlled heavily.

a. Fold your index finger into the palm.
b. Touch the tip of your index finger on the inner ball of your thumb.
c. Touch the ring and middle finger tips with the thumb.
d. Hold the position for 15–20 minutes.
e. Change hands.
f. Repeat daily.

Mudra # 16

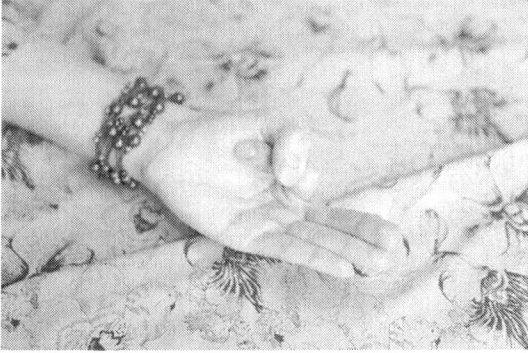

Vayu Mudra

Commonly known as the mudra for wind energy, this position is used to empower chronic complaints like obesity, stress and other fatigue-related ailments of the body and mind. One must strengthen the flow of vayu through the body in order to cut down on weight. The mudra focuses on synchronizing the breathing and biological pattern and clock respectively in the body.

   a. Fold your index finger.
   b. Touch the tip onto the thumb on the inside of your palm.
   c. Now fold your thumb over this gently.
   d. Hold this position for 15–20 minutes.
   e. Change hands.
   f. Continue many times daily.

Mudra # 17

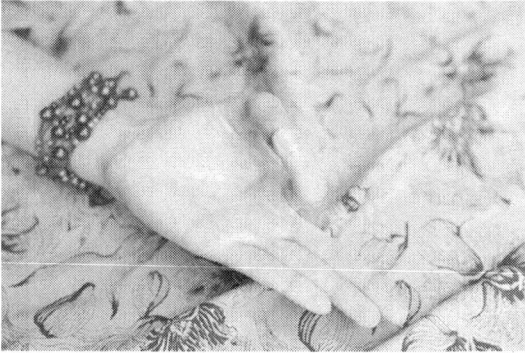

Gyan Mudra

One of the main mudras for the peace of body and mind alike, gyan mudra focuses on relaxing the body in its beginning god health. It helps the mind focus well onto the goal of meditation and losing into meditation.

a. Sit or stand in a comfortable position.
b. Hold your back straight.
c. Hold your chest out.
d. Hold your head high.
e. Rest your hands on your knees, loosened up.
f. Face the palm upwards.
g. Of your right hand, touch the tips of thumb and index finger.
h. Hold your remaining fingers straight out.
i. Parallel their straightness.
j. Now repeat with the other hand.
k. Continue to do 15–20 minute sessions of this mudra three times a day.

Mudra # 18

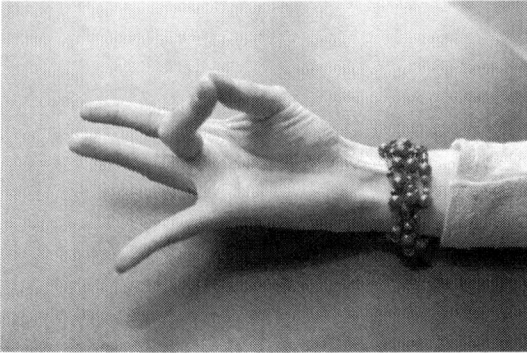

Aakash mudra

Performed to activate the inactive self in our bodies, aakash mudra relies on the power of growing higher thoughts, ideas, detoxifies and enables Extra Sensory Powers (ESP) through burning the inactive physique and mental aches. The mudra also heals uneven counts of heart beats and reduces high blood pressure.

   a. Join the tips of your thumb and middle finger.
   b. Hold the position for 15–20 minutes.
   c. Continue with each hand.
   d. Meditate daily through 6 sessions of aakash mudra.

CHAPTER 6

MUDRAS IV

This chapter enfolds some higher techniques to combat the problem of weight on the body. Mudra power utilizes many techniques of the mind and body to cure and customize the body into good health, hygiene and freedom. These mudras heal hearing aches, ailments and disorders almost instantly.

Mudra # 19

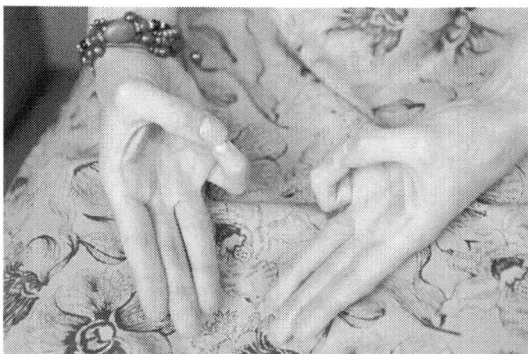

Jal Mudra

Commonly known as the mudra to help the water flow in our body, this mudra helps fight cramps, dehydration, indigestion, scanty semen, hormonal deficiencies and constipation.

    a. Touch the tip of your little fingers against each thumb of each hand.
    b. Now straighten out the rest of your fingers.
    c. Hold the back straight and do breathing exercises for 40–45 minutes.
    d. Meditate the focus to increase that flowing element of the body.
    e. The mudra helps many gastro-intestinal disorders as well aches of the body and mind.
    f. Perform the mudra regularly to achieve weight loss benefits added with great immunity and good health!

Mudra # 20

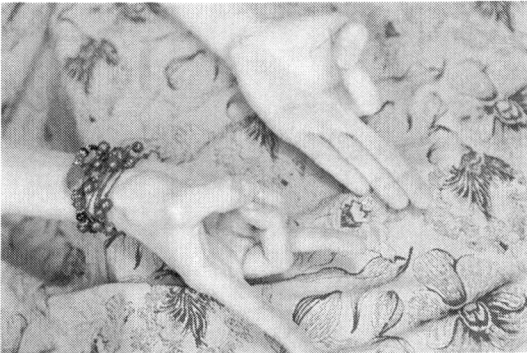

Back Mudra

Commonly known as the mudra to relieve back pain and the aches of the posterior part of the body with mental power, this can also heal mental aches, blocks and insomnia. If you've suddenly cracked your back uneven, do this mudra to aptly resolve the ache. This mudra is also great if you're a worker who is reserved to one or two positions for long hours. Too much stress and obesity can be resolved by this mudra as well. Try to do the mudra in positions that are comforting to your back.

  a. For the right hand: Touch the tips of your thumb, little and middle fingers and point the remaining fingers erect, upwards.
  b. For the left hand: Touch the tip of your index fingernail onto the thumb pad.
  c. Hold both the positions with proper breathing exercise and meditation for 30–40 minutes three times a day.

Mudra # 21

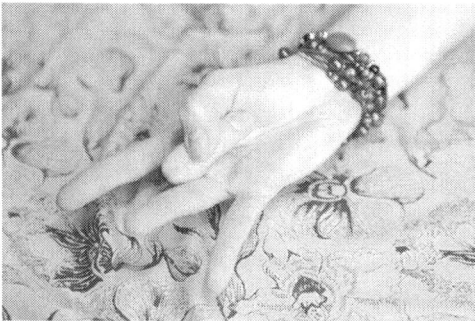

Shunya Mudra

Also known as the mudra for seeking heaven or enlightenment, physique and mind of the celestials, the mudra is focused on curing all sensory aches of the body.

  a. Fold your middle finger onto the ball of your thumb.
  b. Now fold your thumb over this.
  c. Press gently.
  d. Keep your remaining fingers straight upwards.
  e. Hold the position and meditate for 20–30 minutes three times a day.

Mudra # 22

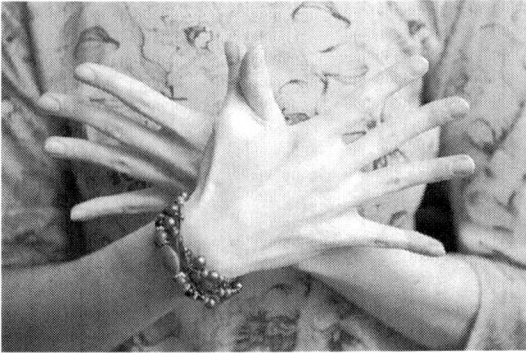

Garuda Mudra

Mudra inspired by the mystical bird, garuda mudra is concerned with the blood circulation, fat deposits and balance of energy in the body and mind. For high blood pressure individuals, do daily once for 4 minutes.

a. Face both your palms open so that your eyes can see them in front of you.
b. Now clasp your thumbs against each other tight.
c. Straighten out the rest of your fingers.
d. Remain in this position for 10 minutes.
e. Now move your hand around other positions and remain for 10 minutes or 10 breathing sessions.
f. Do a few times daily.

CHAPTER 7

CORE MUDRA: SURYA MUDRA: HOW TO AND BENEFITS

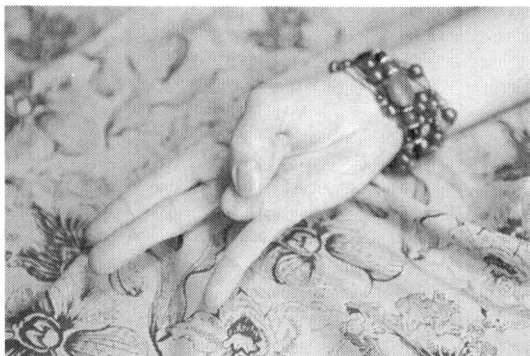

Another element to boost the agni in the body, surya mudra is known to be the most effective or the core mudra for weight loss. This mudra is the core power to de-pressurize various areas of your body in order to increase the fire element in your body. Normally, these elements are suppressed by other greater elements like earth and water. But the fire is the lone omnipotent element that has the power to rage and rise above all.

Method of Performing:

    a. Sit or stand in a comfortable position
    b. Join the tip of your ring fingernail onto the thumb by folding both.
    c. Do it with both the hands.
    d. Do the breathing exercise and continue to meditate and focus.
    e. Focus on firing your body up.
    f. The vision link of agni is enhanced during the performance of this mudra.
    g. Bring gentle pressure to your thumb pad.
    h. Focus higher and continue breathing.
    i. Be in a comfortable posture and position whenever you perform this mudra.

Timing, duration and precautions:

Daily do this mudra for 40–45 minutes in 3 sessions each or 9 sessions. This is a mudra that can be performed to charge your energy and fire for the body at any hour, but early morning, alongside the sun, surya mudra gains more power as the name of the mudra, from Sanskrit, translates to sun in English. Afternoon is an ideal time as well, but morning and sunset is also powerful.

One of the most important things to keep in mind is the over-heating aspect of your body due to the performance of this mudra. One should perform this mudra in regular sessions and take care never to burn it all out of the mind and body.

Effects and Benefits:

As mentioned before, the core mudra, surya mudra, has many mesmerizing positive effects to the body and mind. One of the ancient components of ancient Indian and Buddhist culture and secrets, surya mudra has been known to be the cure for many ailments.

The mudra helps boost the metabolism of the body into making it an active and healthy body. It also provides immunity against the common cold and fevers. If you are intent on losing weight effectively through mudra, make sure you perform all the other mudras and keep yourself in good shape. The mudra gives a power to enhance, enrich and neutralize the temperature of the body as well as strengthen all weaker sections of the body and mind.

Surya mudra proves to be healthy and an elixir to obese people as this effectively sheds weight. Post-pregnancy flab as well as genetic pieces of immovable rock-fat can also vanish with the routine practice of surya mudra. Make sure you follow a lifestyle that fits in with the peace, calmness and temper of your enlightened spirituality, enriched physique and uplifted mentality.

CHAPTER 8

ISSUES OF WEIGHT LOSS THROUGH MUDRAS

As mentioned in the previous chapters, the power of mudras comes along with a strict routine and biological training of your body and its will. There arises many issues throughout the phase of mudra training as this power is supported solely by your own power of discipline and care for your body. When the methods are improper and irregular, there can arise many problems, some of which are:

a. Overheating of the body: As the previous chapter clearly explained, it is within the performer's sense to ritualize and regulate the dormant side of the body to fire up instantly with the power of mudras. However, the point is to follow a discipline alongside the mudra as well. If you simply perform the mudras for several minutes a day randomly and unevenly, there is a clear chance your body and mind will catch fire as well.

b. Oversleeping: Another important effect of improper training of mudra power without apt articulation, charge or focus, oversleeping becomes the comfort. A lazy body also feels exhaustion out of the greed of comfort or luxury. A person tends to become exhausted with all the wrong focus and blocked charging.

c. Hyperactivity: This is a direct result of improper mudra training. As the body trains to metabolize more and activates the years' old innards, it is time for the body to command it to work instantly.

d. Perpetually elevated dose of positivity: This aforementioned hyperactivity results in a perpetually awakened dose of positivity that is impossible to control, eject or emit. One must train properly in order to reap the right effects. Altered effects can do a certain degree of damage to everything connected to the central body.

e. Frustration and Nihilism: The effect of all of the above combined is what results as frustration and nihilism. A man grows frustrated out of mishandling or improperly mediating. This causes a strong nihilism of seeing no colors, oasis or rain.

One must train properly in order to be good at performing mudra power for healing and weight loss mechanisms.

Conclusion

With all these tips, guidelines and issues of mudra power for weight loss being said, it is within one's own individual right to decide on how to crop the way of living. Practicing mudra power religiously for 3 hours daily and moving back to a lifestyle full of ash, smoke and stings is definitely not the way mudra power is practiced. All of this adds to the unhygienic activation of mudra power, which can then result in damaging realities to your one present concrete reality.

One must always learn to abide by the discipline as per the teachings when cultivating the power of mudras and such.

It is within our own powers to regulate and help ourselves to healing and betterment. For weight loss, mudra power can help you immensely and instantly if you're one with discipline and positivity or want to have positivity in your life. Mudra power will grant you positivity, confidence, conviction, worth and enhanced potential of your own unique abilities.

Good Luck!

Book 2

23 MUDRAS FOR SPIRITUAL HEALING

TABLE OF CONTENTS

Chapter 1. Introduction to the mudras 39

Chapter 2. The hands that heal 43

Chapter 3. How to practice mudras 45

Chapter 4. 23 mudras for spiritual healing 48

Chapter 5. Mudra and pranayama 73

Chapter 6. Mudra and meditation 75

Chapte 7. Conclusion 76

INTRODUCTION TO THE MUDRAS

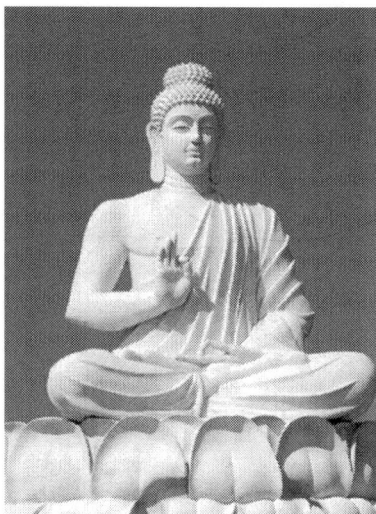

Lord Buddha

"He who practices mudras does not die, nor does he degenerate. He does not fear fire, water or air."

—Gheranda samhita 3/98

With eyes half-closed, sitting cross-legged, poised in grace and a halo around the head, the mere sight of a statue of Lord Buddha enthralls us, fills us with compassion, love, and tranquility. Lord Buddha sits in a state of meditation. Ever thought what is that peculiar gesture of hand he always appears to assume in every embodiment? This is known as the mudra. Other than Buddha, almost every Hindu deity and god is depicted in one or the other mudra. For long, this art and science was considered to be the right of the priests and sages. People were advised to practice the mudras secretly. But the mudras are no more confined to a particular sect of people and anyone can practice them at a place and time best suited to them.

UNDERSTANDING THE MUDRAS

Mudra is a Sanskrit word. Its literal meaning is seal, mark, posture, or pose. A pose or gesture assumed by the body that helps redirect and channelize the energy flow in such a way that the energy produces physical, mental, and spiritual healing is known as the mudra. Postures of hand, postures of body (asanas), and locks (bandhas) are included in the mudras. Some are pure gestures of hand while the others are a combination of hand gestures and breathing exercises.

How would a man have communicated before he could read, write, and speak? Before the advent of language, man was already using the mudras, but he understood the importance of the mudras some time later. We all use gestures to express our feelings. The ancient sages thought that a vice versa relation was also possible. That is, we can control our mood, feelings, body, mind, and soul by mastering the art of mudras. They researched for ages and developed numerous mudras that were beneficial for the body and life. Hathyog Pradipika by the Patanjali, Siva Samhita and Gherand Samhita are the earliest scriptures available that contain the description of the mudras, how to do them, and their benefits. Buddhism is also replete with the ancient texts on mudras. Similar forms of mudras are found around the world with different names such as yin in China and in in Japan. Mudras have been described in two contexts in ancient Indian texts. One is natya mudra and the other is yoga mudra. Natya mudras are the graceful gestures employed in various classical dance moves and resemble the yoga mudras.

In Hathyog Pradipika and in Siva Samhita, 10 yoga mudras are described. And in Gherand Samhita, 25 yoga mudras are described. According to the other school of thought, there are 12 types of mudras, 10 types of mahamudras and three types of bandhas. Here we discuss the yoga mudras that are useful in spiritual healing.

During conversation with the Goddess Chanda Kapali, Gherand in the Gherand Samhita speaks highly of the mudras,

"O Chanda! What more shall I tell thee? In brief, there is nothing on the earth like the mudras that help achieve the enlightenment."

—Gherand Samhita 3/100

He says that besides being the foe of the decay and death, the mudras destroy all the diseases. Cough, asthma, enlargement of spleen, leprosy, and all sorts of ailments are alleviated. The metabolic energy and the digestive power of the man improve. And the mudras ultimately give happiness.

41

THE MUDRAS AND THE KUNDALINI YOGA

The mudras are also a tool to awaken the kundalini as is said by The Patanjali:

> "To awaken the Goddess (The kundalini) who sleeps at the entrance of the Brahma Dwara (the great door), the mudras should be practiced well."

> —Hath Yoga Pradipika 3/5

The kundalini yoga, also known as the laya yoga is considered to be one of the best to generate more power with stability within oneself. The yoga is based on arousing the kundalini. The kundalini is considered to be the snake-like energy lying spirally. The aim is to straighten it and make it travel through the spinal cord to the highest center, i.e., the brain. The mudras act as the specific points and meridians, which when pressed help the arising energy. Recent studies also support the fact that touching the specific points on a hand stimulates specific areas of the brain. Lothar, a well-known expert of kundalini yoga says:

"In this respect, Kundalini Yoga assumes that every area of the hand forms a reflex zone for an associated part of the body and the brain. In this way, we can consider the hands to be a mirror for our body and our mind."

Let us together unleash the power of the breathtaking mudra yoga. Before we start practicing, let us peep into the types of yoga mudras.

CHAPTER 2

THE HANDS THAT HEAL

The face is the mirror of the mind. This is the generally accepted fact. Did you know the hand is the mirror of the body? It is now a scientifically proven fact that all the nerves of the body terminate in the hands. Thus, both the hands are connected to each part of the body and a desired effect can be achieved by identifying and pressurizing the connecting points on the hand. The hand is considered to be connected more to the brain and the spinal cord than any part of the body. Calmness of mind brings about the calmness of hand and vice versa. The mudras are therefore a pathway to achieve an increased awareness and hassle-free awakening.

According the Ayurvedic concept, the five fingers represent the five basic elements of the body. The five elements with their respective finger are:

The thumb: the fire element
The index finger: the air element
The middle finger: the sky/the vacuum element
The ring finger: the earth element
The little finger: water element

According to the kundalini yoga, the chakras are also connected to the hand. The five fingers representing the five chakras are:

The thumb: the solar plexus chakra
The index finger: the heart chakra
The middle finger: the throat chakra
The ring finger: the root chakra
The little finger: the sacral chakra

Several points have now been identified that are connected to different diseases such as high blood pressure, asthma, heart attack, diarrhea, etc.

Different mudras include making a seal or a ring of different fingers causing different elements to activate which brings about a cascade of changes inside the body. Keeping in view the representations of different fingers, own mudras can also be developed to suit one self.

CHAPTER 3

HOW TO PRACTICE MUDRAS

The best part of practicing the mudras is that they do not need strict measures to be followed prior practice. The mudras can be practiced anywhere and at any time. Yet if a few guidelines are kept in consideration, the effect can be increased manifold.

Mudras are basically gestures. So you need to keep your hands relaxed. The fingers tend to curl up after some time. So you can use the other hand to keep the fingers steady. With practice, you will gradually become habitual of keeping the hand in position for longer durations.

The fingers should touch each other gently and a moderate pressure should be applied. Mild pressure will not be able to bring about any effect whereas excessive pressure will bring about fatigue to the muscles of the fingers. Hence, a moderate pressure is desirable.

WHEN TO PRACTICE THE MUDRAS

While commuting to the work in the train or dozing off during break at work, after waking up, or before sleep the mudras can be practiced anywhere with relative ease. But if a time slot is allotted to practicing the mudras, it would result better. The best time is during morning hours when the mind and body are peaceful. At that time the mudras can be supplemented with various yoga postures and meditation.

WHERE TO PRACTICE THE MUDRAS

The best place is a serene vicinity with fresh air and a soothing environment where you can concentrate while practicing the mudras. Otherwise, a closed room with the minimum scope of disturbance is also useful. Other than these, the mudras can be practiced anywhere.

POSITION FOR PRACTICING MUDRAS

When you are practicing the mudras at your workplace, then they can be practiced in the position you usually assume at the workplace. Only you have to take care that the body remains straight and relaxed. There must be no tension in the body and you must be very comfortable. If you are sitting on a chair, ensure that you sit straight and your feet touch the ground. The cushion must be soft enough to let you sit in a relaxed posture.

If you are practicing the mudras at your home, you can sit in meditative positions. Sitting cross-legged or half cross-legged, the lotus posture, or other poses of yoga may be assumed. For this keep the following points in mind:

- Sit straight. Straighten your back. Both the flexion and hyperextension of the back creates early fatigue in the muscles of the back. So a position where a perfect balance between the two is maintained should be searched for. This is the position of least fatigability and you will be able to endure prolonged sitting.

- Let your hands rest on the knees.
- Breathe gently. Observe the calm flow of the air in and out of the nostrils. Imagine the air inflating the lungs like a balloon and deflating as you breathe out.
- Relax your whole body. Ensure that any ailing part of the body is addressed before you sit for practicing the mudras. The body must slip into rest mode.

Other than this, mudras can also be practiced while standing, walking, or in a lying down position. If you are standing, maintain the posture that is the most comfortable. Keeping your back and neck straight, letting shoulders fall backwards, arms by the side, and legs a few centimeters apart makes the most comfortable standing position. And lying down on your back with the legs at some distance and feet falling outwards makes a good position too. In a nutshell, whatever position you are in, you must keep your body straight and in symmetrical alignment. Yet do take care not to make it too stiff.

DURATION FOR THE MUDRAS

The duration for practicing mudras depends on the type of mudra and the purpose of practicing mudras. The range is from 3 to 45 minutes for an individual mudra.

CHAPTER 4

23 MUDRAS FOR SPIRITUAL HEALING

As has been said before, there are numerous mudras that have been described in ancient texts. There are many others that have been added to the vast collection of the mudras for ages. Some are similar while some are completely different mudras. A few mudras are formed by a single hand while there are some where two hands are needed to complete the form of the mudra. There are some mudras that involve the whole body. Although all the mudras are beneficial in spiritual growth, there are some that have a special effect on spiritual healing. We will lay our focus only on the mudras that are involved in spiritual healing. Here are the 23 mudras helpful in healing of body, mind, and spirit.

MUDRA 1: GYAN MUDRA

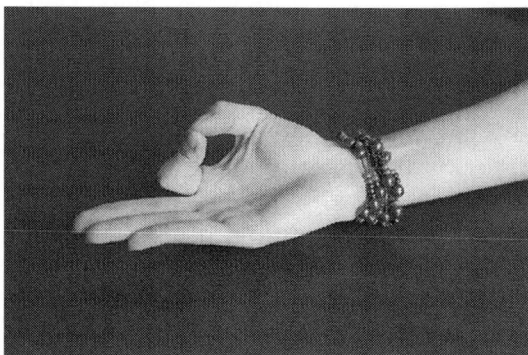

Description: Gyan is a Sanskrit word meaning knowledge and wisdom. The main purpose of the gyan mudra is to help achieve spiritual growth and enlightenment. It is mostly practiced during breathing exercises and meditation.

Method: Touch the tip of the index finger with the tip of the thumb and extend the other three fingers. Place the hand on the thigh facing towards the sky. This is gyan mudra.

This mudra can be done during meditation in the lotus pose or semi-lotus pose. Close your eyes and focus on your breath while keeping the hands in gyan mudra. You may also chant OM every time you exhale.

Time: 5–45 minutes. Either it can be done once a day for 45 minutes or for 5 minutes three times a day.

Usefulness: It is the foremost mudra that is both simple and useful in spiritual healing. It helps the light of knowledge pierce the darkness of ignorance. It is the mudra for enlightenment.

Physical effects: It increases the vayu content in the body. Thus it enhances the function of the nervous, the endocrine, and the musculoskeletal systems. Any sort of disorders caused by dysfunctioning of the nervous system, hypo secretions of the endocrine disorders, and muscular disorders are alleviated by this mudra.

This should be practiced moderately by the people of vata predominant prakriti (nature).

It also fills in energy and enthusiasm in the person. As the name goes, it incites the brain to learn new things and indulge into exciting adventures.

MUDRA 2: CHIN MUDRA

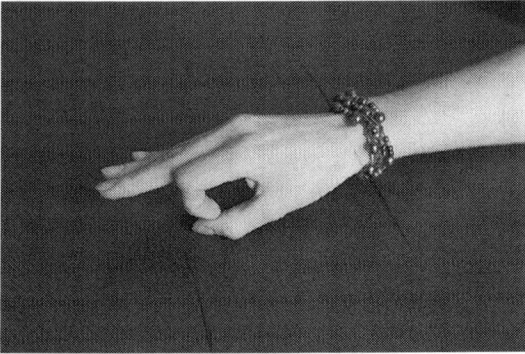

Description: Chin in Sanskrit means consciousness. It is the mudra that helps awaken the divine consciousness. It is the other form of gyan mudra. Some consider it the gyan mudra itself while others consider it a separate entity. However, it is identical to the gyan mudra in position and only a little difference in their effects exists.

The thumb represents the supreme self, the index finger represents the self, the middle represents the ego, the ring finger represents illusion, and the little one is related to karma. So, the mudra helps unite the individual self with the supreme self while setting aside the ego, illusion, and karma.

Method: The tip of the thumb touches the tip of the index finger. The hand does not face the sky; the hand faces the ground. This is the chin mudra.

Time: Similar to the gyan mudra.

Usefulness: It helps increase the concentration power during meditation and improves your sleep pattern. It is also said to have beneficial effects on low backache, improves energy, and reduces lethargy.

MUDRA 3: LING MUDRA

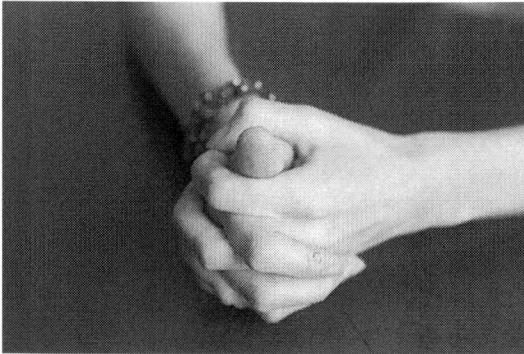

Description: Ling is the Sanskrit word meaning phallus, i.e. the male genital organ. This mudra is also known as the upright mudra. It is very helpful in calming the mind. Excessive use of the mudra may sometimes result in sluggishness.

Method: Clasp both the hands and interlock the fingers. Touch the thumb that is on the top with the tip of the index finger of the same hand so that the thumb of the other hand lies encircled by the ring formed by the thumb and the index finger of the other hand. Keep the encircled thumb straight. This is ling mudra.

Time: This may be practiced up to 15 minutes.

Physical effects: It increases the heat and fire quotient of the body—that is, it increases pitta. It is a good remedy for coughing and colds. It helps reduce the extra fat in the body and decreases the kapha in the body.

MUDRA 4: ATAMANJALI MUDRA

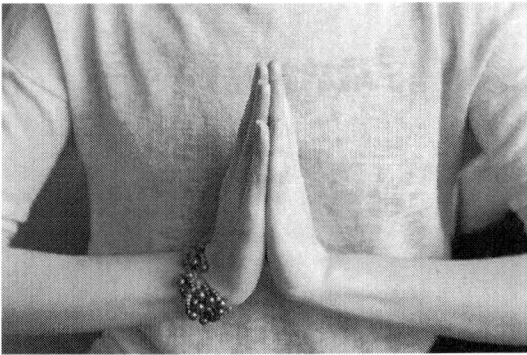

Description: This is the gesture commonly followed in eastern nations during prayer and also when greeting people. Anjali is a Sanskrit word meaning "salutation with reverence." "Atma" denotes "the self." Thus the atmanjali means respecting the self.

The joining of the two palms is said to establish a connection between the two hemispheres of the brain. It is like completing the circuit that originates from the brain, passes through the one hand to the other, and finally back to the brain.

Method: Bring the two hands together close to your heart and join the two palms and fingers with each other. Press the two hands against each other gently so that the space between the two palms remains hollow.

Time: You may remain in the position as long as you are in prayer or in meditation. Or it can be done for 10–15 minutes.

Usefulness: The mudra plays a very important role in relieving stress and helps achieve more focus and concentration in meditation and in daily life too. It also maintains the balance between the left and the right hemispheres. It also brings peace and harmony in life.

MUDRA 5: PRAN MUDRA

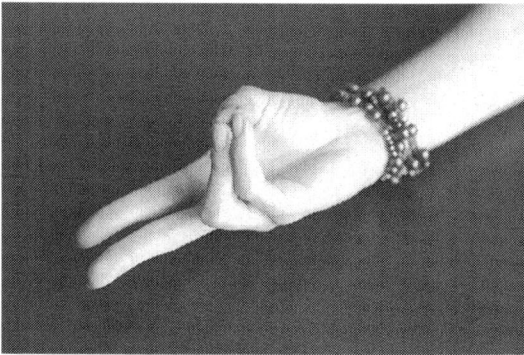

Description: "Pran" is life. "Pran vayu" is the part of "vayu" that is the vital force without which the person is a dead body. The manifestation part of the "pran vayu" is the breath. The minute the breath stops, a person ceases to live. The mudra for this vayu is pran vayu.

Method: Touch the tip of the ring finger and the little finger with the thumb. Extend the index finger and the middle finger. Do it with each hand. This is known as the pran mudra.

Time: 15 minutes

Usefulness: This mudra is the elixir of life. It increases the vitality, strengthens the immune system, and improves the immune system. It helps in fatigue and low resistance to diseases. It helps improve general condition in chronic debilitating diseases.

Emotions that depress the mood are effectively controlled. It is also an amplifier of the effects of other mudras and is done in association with them. It is a very important mudra for spiritual growth.

MUDRA 6: APAN MUDRA

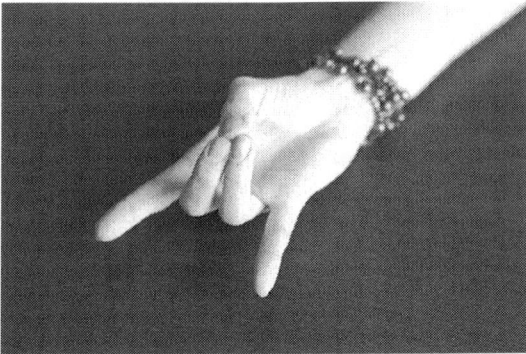

Description: Apan vayu is another type of vayu found in the body. It is also known as the mrit sanjeevani mudra as it was considered that it saved the life of a person having a heart attack.

Method: Touch the tip of the thumb with the tips of the middle finger and the ring finger. Extend the other two fingers. This is apan mudra.

Time: 10–15 minutes

Usefulness: This mudra has a very beneficial effect on the heart. A person affected with a heart disease must practice this mudra.

The mudra pertains to the apan vayu. Hence, all the functions of apan vayu are improved. The gastric motility improves and constipation and indigestion are relieved. The wastes of the body are eliminated properly and the body is relieved of the toxins.

It also promotes confidence and self-esteem.

MUDRA 7: VAYU MUDRA

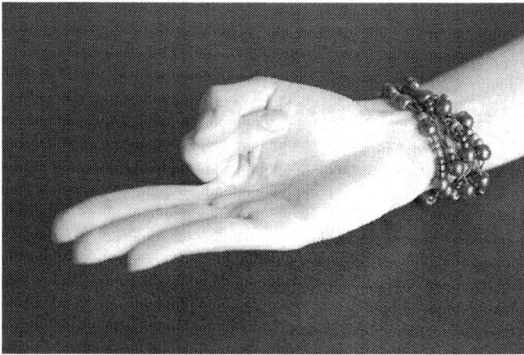

Description: Vayu is a Sanskrit word for the air. The vayu in the body regulates various functions of the body. The nervous system is chiefly associated with the vayu.

Method: Curl the index finger and place the thumb on it. Gently press the finger by the thumb. Extend the other fingers. Do this with each hand. This is the vayu mudra.

Time: 15 minutes

Usefulness: This mudra is useful in "vayu" related problems such as nervous disorders, paralysis, joint pains, tremors, etc.

The mudra is beneficial in stress, anxiety, sleeplessness and restlessness.

MUDRA 8: SHUNYA MUDRA

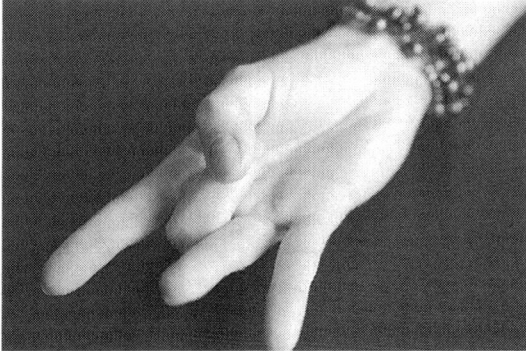

Description: Shunya in Sanskrit means vacuum, nothingness, or the sky. It is also the word for zero. Shunya is one of the five basic elements that make up the body. This mudra is for balancing this element.

Method: Curl the middle finger and place the thumb on it and gently press the middle finger by the thumb. This is known as shunya mudra.

Time: 15 minutes

Usefulness: As the shunya or the sky element is associated with the function of hearing, all the disorders related to hearing are relieved by this mudra.

This mudra also plays a role in spiritual awakening. The person feels connected to the god in the initial stages of meditation. This mudra gives the person eternal bliss.

MUDRA 9: PRITHIVI MUDRA

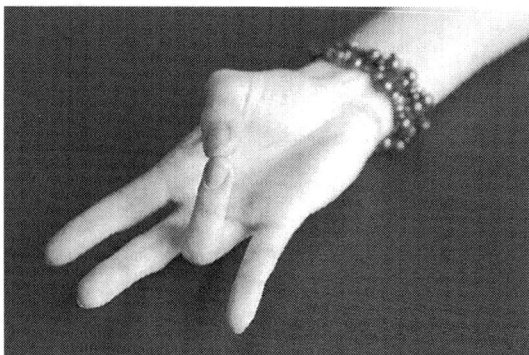

Description: Prithivi is the fifth basic element in the body. This mudra decreases the fire element in the body and increases the kapha or the prithivi element.

Method: Touch the tip of the thumb with the tip of the ring finger. Extend the rest of the fingers. Do this with each hand. This is the prithivi mudra.

Time: 15 minutes a day

Usefulness: As this mudra increases the prithivi element of the body, it increases the strength of the bones, the muscles, the tendons, the ligaments, and various other structures. It also improves the disorders of nose and smell.

It also helps boost confidence

MUDRA 10: VARUNA MUDRA

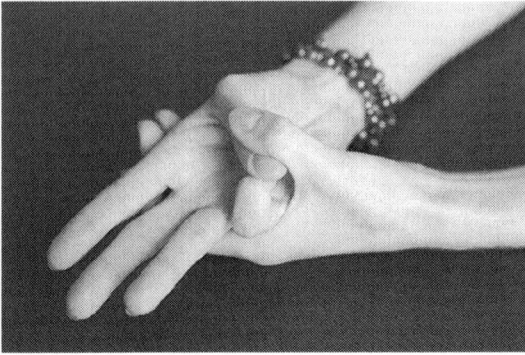

Description: Varuna means water. This mudra relates to the water element of the body.

Method: Touch the tip of the little finger with the ball of the thumb of the same hand. Extend the index, the middle, and the ring finger. Keep this hand on the other hand at a right angle to each other. Put the thumb of the other hand on the circle formed by the little finger and the thumb of the other hand. Press the thumb on it. Let the rest of the fingers of the other hand encircle the first hand. This is the varuna mudra.

Time: 45 minutes

Usefulness: The mudra is useful in dispelling the diseases which occur due to water deficiency in the body. It improves the turgor of the skin imparting its beauty. It purifies the blood by removing the toxins from the body.

This mudra also helps in improving taste and curing diseases related to taste.

MUDRA 11: PUSHAN MUDRA

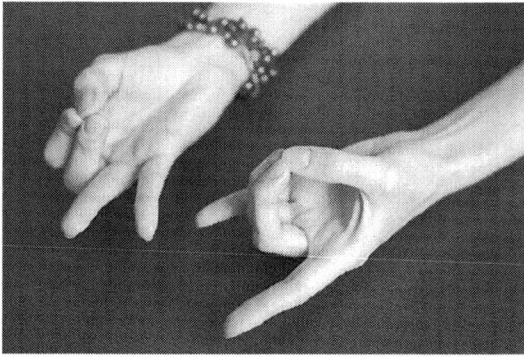

Description: This mudra is related the sun. He is considered to be the god of nourishment and fulfillment.

Method: Touch the tip of your index finger and the middle finger with the thumb and extend the ring finger and the little finger. This is the mudra for the right hand. Alternatively, the little finger and the ring finger can be touched with the thumb while the index finger and the middle finger remain extended.

Now touch the tip of your middle finger and the ring finger with the tip of the thumb and extend the index finger and the little finger. This is the pose to be attained by the left hand. This is known as the pushan mudra.

Time: 5 minutes

Usefulness: As is clear from the description above, this mudra is related to digestion. The digestion process improves and hence nutrition is maintained. This mudra can be performed after having a meal to have a good effect on digestion.

MUDRA 12: HAKINI MUDRA

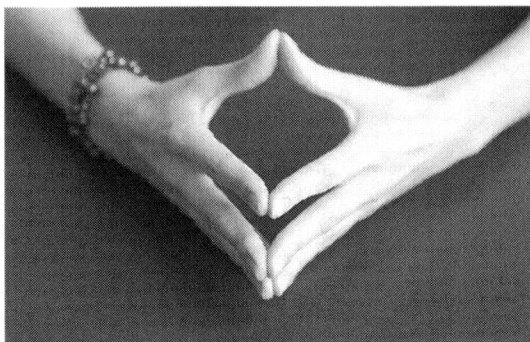

Description: Hakini is the supreme power associated with the sixth chakra that lies in the forehead. It is related to the memorization and recalling power of the brain.

Method: Touch the fingertips of one hand with the corresponding fingertips of the other hand. Four fingertips and the tip of the thumb of each hand must be included.

Time: 5-15 minutes

Usefulness: This is the best mudra for memory. If you want to memorize something you can sit with your hands in this mudra, close your eyes, and memorize. It is also helpful in recalling something you have forgotten. For this you have to follow simple meditation steps. Close the eyes, keep your hands in hakini mudra, and take your awareness to your breath. The forgotten memory will eventually dawn upon you.

It also improves the coordination between the right and left hemispheres of the brain.

MUDRA 13: SHANKH MUDRA

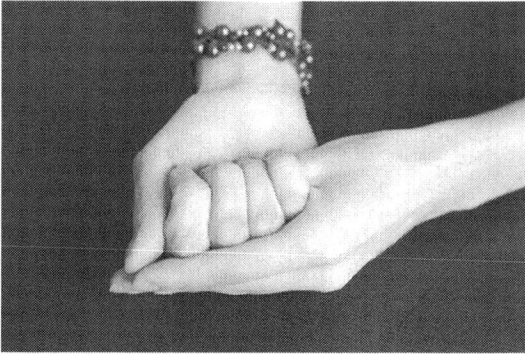

Description: Shankh is the Sanskrit name for conch shell. It holds an important place in religious ceremonies in India.

Method: Clench the fist of the left hand. Now extend the thumb. Extend the other hand and keep the clenched fist on the left hand in such a way that the thumb touches the middle finger of the other hand. Hold the mudra in this position in front of the sternum.

Time: 15 minutes

Usefulness: The mudra is very beneficial in bringing peace and calmness. It helps immerse the vastness of the universe in the self.

It soothes the respiratory system. The breathing deepens and becomes calm.

MUDRA **14:** SURABHI MUDRA

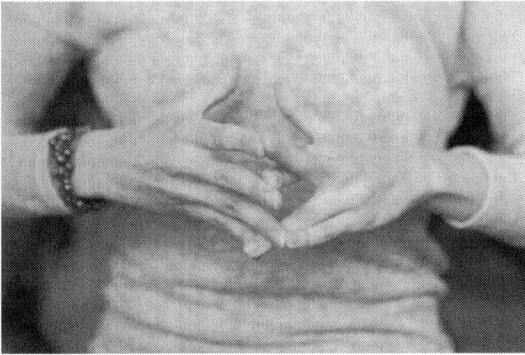

Description: It is also known as the kamdhenu mudra. Kamdhenu is the mythological cow. It is believed that the person practicing the mudra is able to attain all his wishes through the wish granting kamdhenu cow.

Method: Touch the index finger of the left hand with the middle finger of the right hand and do the same with the middle finger of the left hand and the index finger of the right hand. Simultaneously, touch the little finger of the left hand with the finger of the right hand and vice versa. Extend the two thumbs and they remain free. This mudra is known as the surabhi mudra.

Time: 15 minutes

Usefulness: It is known to be one of the most powerful mudras as it helps utilize the power of all the five elements. It works on the nabhi (navel) chakra and helps improve digestion.

MUDRA 15: KUNDALINI MUDRA

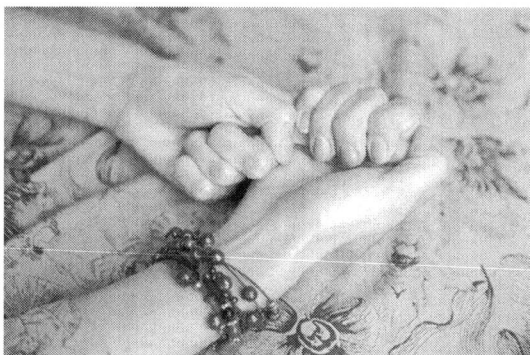

Description: This mudra is the mudra of sexuality and kindles the sexual energy of the person.

Method: Clench both hands into loose fists. Place the index finger of the right hand into the fist of the left hand. Cover the tip of the index finger of the right hand by the thumb of the left hand. Keep the hands in front of your abdomen. This is the kundalini mudra.

Time: 5–10 minutes

Usefulness: This chakra is helpful in rejuvenating the capability of reproduction and regeneration. This is also the place for creativity. Creativity, too, increases by this mudra. When you are creative, you are in meditation.

MUDRA 16: GANESHA MUDRA

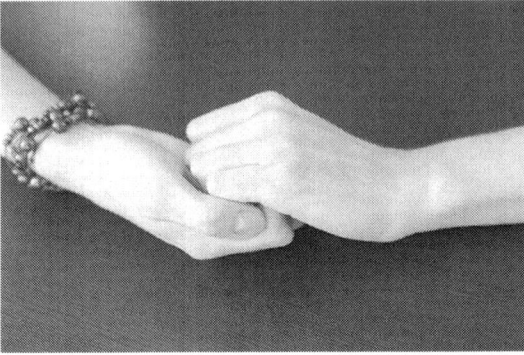

Description: Lord Ganesha is the first lord that is beckoned before the inauguration of any event or ceremony in Hindu religion. Any deed cannot be completed without the permission of Lord Ganesha. The mudra of his name is thus a very powerful mudra which is very beneficial for the heart and for stepping into the world of spirituality.

Method: Clasp the hands in such a way that the fingers of each hand lie in the palm of the other hand and hook the fingers of the other hand.

Keep the mudra in front of your chest and pull both the arms towards the opposite side keeping the fingers hooked.

Time: 15 minutes

Usefulness: This is very helpful in strengthening heart muscles and giving relief in cardiac ailments.

MUDRA 17: KUBERA MUDRA

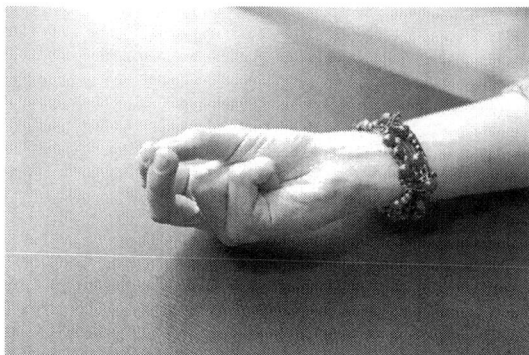

Description: Kubera is the god of wealth. The mudra is about visualizing the goals and achieving them.

Method: Touch the tip of the thumb with the tips of the index finger and the middle finger simultaneously. Curl the ring finger and the little finger and embed them into the center of the palm. This is known as the kubera mudra.

Time: 5–15 minutes

Usefulness: Visualizing your goals and imagining that you are already in the possession of your desired object or situation along with the mudra takes you to your goal.

In addition, this mudra has been found to be beneficial treating sinus problems.

MUDRA 18: RUDRA MUDRA

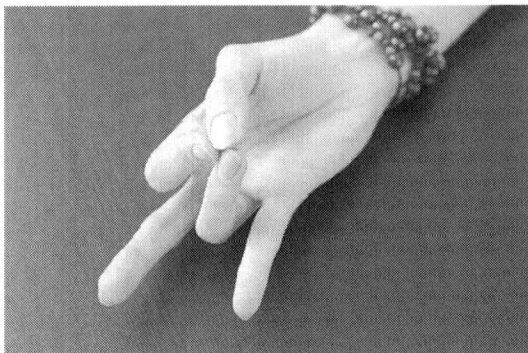

Description: Rudra is the name of Lord Shiva who is the destroyer and the transformer. The mudra helps clear and make space for new things. It clears the mind and makes way for greater concentration power.

Method: Touch the tip of the thumb with the tip of the index finger and the ring finger simultaneously. Extend the middle finger and the little finger. These fingers tend to curl up, so you will have to put in extra effort to keep them relatively straight. Try not to put excessive strain on your hand muscles.

Time: 5 minutes daily will suffice. The mudra may be repeated three times a day if possible.

Usefulness: It maintains the homeostasis in the body. It maintains the balance of the body. It maintains the blood pressure and regulates respiration.

MUDRA 19: KALESHVARA MUDRA

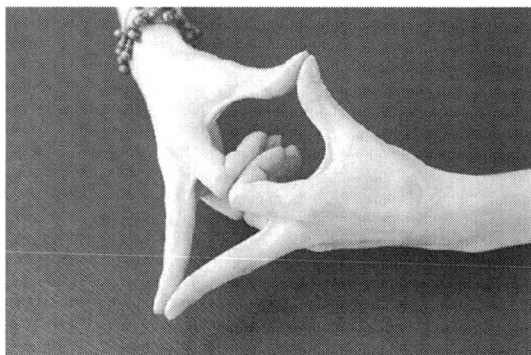

Description: The kaleshvara is the Lord of Time. The mudra is helpful if you want to adapt and improve with time. It helps you change what is embedded deep in your character.

Method: Touch the tips of the middle fingers of both hands. Then touch the tips of the two thumbs. Bring the rest of the fingers close together to touch the proximal joints of the corresponding fingers. Place your hand in front of the chest in such a way that the joined tips of the thumbs point towards the chest.

Time: It can be practiced for 15 minutes per day

Usefulness: It helps make you more peaceful and put away conflicting thoughts.

It helps if you want to change for good and do away with the harmful habits that have plagued you. If you want to shun smoking, drinking, or any type of drug abuse, this mudra is for you.

MUDRA 20: SHIVA LINGA MUDRA

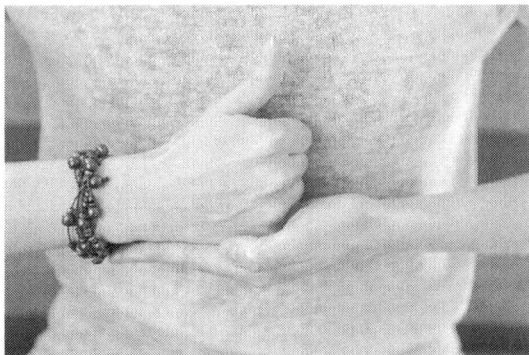

Description: Shiva is a god in Hindu mythology and is considered to be the destructive and transformative force. Things must be destroyed to create new ones. Thus this force is maintained by this mudra.

Method: Bring your left hand close to your abdomen and turn the palm upwards towards the sky. The hand must be in bowl shape. Clench your right hand into a fist. Release and straighten the thumb to let it point towards the sky. Keep the right hand in this position on the left hand. This is shiva linga mudra.

Time: 10–15 minutes.

Usefulness: The mudra fills the reservoir of energy in the body, fights against depression, and gives excitement.

MUDRA 21: DHYANI MUDRA

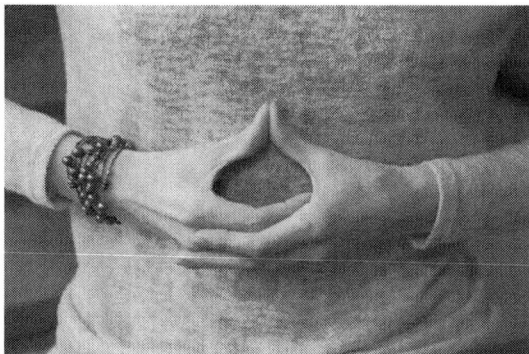

Description: This is the mudra of meditation. While meditating, the person sits in meditation pose and this mudra is assumed. The negativities are released by the open hands and the hands become receptacle to the subtle energies of the universe.

It is said that one can achieve peace and tranquility just by looking at the mudra being performed by an adept.

Method: Sit in lotus or semi-lotus posture. Place the right hand on the midline of the crossed leg with the palm facing upwards and the hand in a bowl shape. Place the left hand on the right hand in similar form. Now touch the tips of both thumbs. This is the dhyani mudra.

Time: 5 minutes

Usefulness: This helps the mind clear away all the disturbing thoughts and become centered.

MUDRA 22: LOTUS MUDRA

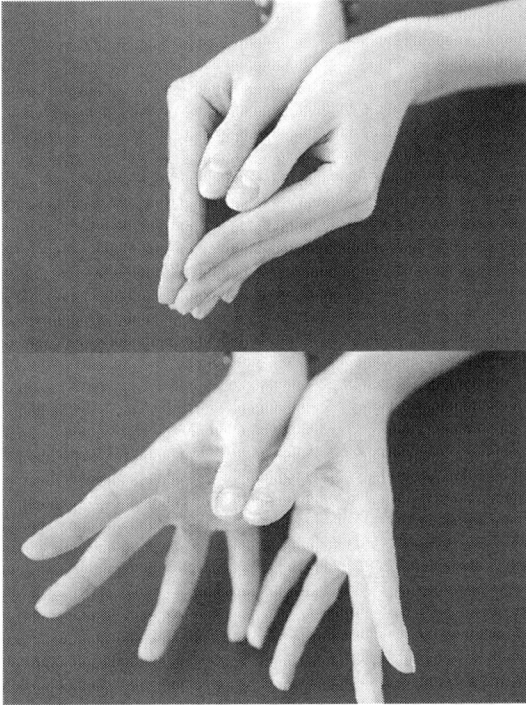

Description: As the name suggests, the resultant mudra that the two hands assume resembles the lotus flower. The hands are kept in front of the heart and represent the heart opening up to the world of spirituality. It lets go of the feelings that are undesirable and embraces the purity and divinity.

Method: Bring both hands in front of your posture and join the hands as in atmanjali mudra. But do not touch the whole area of the fingers nor place the palms with each other as in atmanjali mudra. Instead, touch only the fingertips and the tips of the thumbs. This is the bud of the lotus.

Now gently open the finger-bud and let it bloom into a full grown flower. Expand the fingers to their fullest. Take a breath in while closing the finger-bud and breathe out while opening the flower.

Time: 5–10 minutes.

Usefulness: This mudra is very useful in generating affection, love, and unconditional love in the heart. It helps us socialize with others and share our love, joy, and sorrows.

This mudra helps activate the anahata chakra in the heart and bring out compassion.

MUDRA 23: NAGA MUDRA

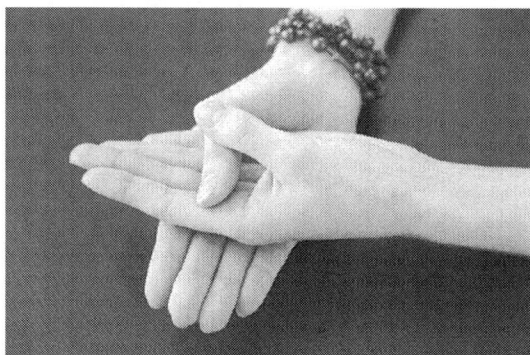

Description: Naga stands for the serpent and the serpent represents strength. The aim is to fight the distractions on the path to salvation with the mighty strength of the serpent.

Method: Keep your one hand over the other in a way that the two hands are at right angles to each other. Cross the two thumbs similarly. Keep your hands close to the chest in this mudra. This is known as the naga mudra.

Time: 15 minutes

Usefulness: The mudra is useful for a deep insight. It clears the mind of disturbing thoughts and imparts the person wisdom.

It is also helpful in relieving worries.

MUDRA AND PRANAYAMA

Pranayama is made up of two words: "prana" and "ayama." The meaning of which is, "that which channelizes the vital force in the body through a varied number of breathing techniques." The pranayama includes the exercises that are classified on the basis of difference in speed, pattern, depth, and muscles used in respiration. These biophysical changes in breathing patterns results in a change in oxygen and carbon dioxide levels in the body triggering various mechanisms in the body that ultimately cleanse the body and the mind.

THE MUDRAS FOR PRANAYAMA

The mudras are used in conjunction with the pranayama. The mudras lay a synergistic effect on the healing properties of pranayama and take the person towards a higher awakening. The mudras channelize the flow of prana—the vital force through the body which is kindled by the pranayama. The mudras commonly used with the pranayama are: the chin mudra, the gyan mudra, the chinmayi mudra, the adi mudra, the dhyaani mudra, and the pran vayu mudra. The chinmayi mudra is similar to the chin mudra, but the three fingers are not extended and instead embedded in the palm as is done in the fist. The adi mudra is nothing but a loose fist. Others have been described earlier.

CHAPTER 6

MUDRA AND MEDITATION

Meditation is the last step of yoga. It leads towards the unification with the God. It is the way to live steadily through the waxing and waning of life. A lot has happened before and a lot is happening right now. All of it gets stored in the brain. The brain has assumed more of the role of recycle bin as it has accumulated trash over past few years. Meditation is the method to clear the dust and it will stand guard against the unnecessary thoughts and memories from entering into the brain. The mudras are the helpers of meditation.

MUDRAS FOR MEDITATION

As has been described earlier, the mudras direct the energy flow while meditating and help the rise of the kundalini force. The mudras used in meditation are: the gyan mudra, the dhyaani mudra, the chin mudra, the chinmayi mudra, the shunya mudra, the vayu mudra, the pran mudra, the prithivi mudra, and many others.

Practice the mudras while meditating and experience even more wonderful effects.

Conclusion

When you grow spiritually, all the dimensions of life improve. Physical, mental, and emotional disturbances are effectively countered. Yoga and meditation are the pathways of spiritual growth. The mudras hold a paramount place in yoga. When coupled with meditation and various yoga postures, the mudras help grow at a better and faster pace.

Close your eyes and imagine all the things you want in life. Now ask a question for yourself: Why do you need all the things? The answer is simple. We all want our lives to be happy, calm, and peaceful. A peaceful state of mind is only achieved by strengthening the inner self. The mudras help attain the awakening, the knowledge, and the enlightenment. The ultimate truth transcends. Therefore, practice the mudras described above and traverse the path to eternal bliss and complete joy.

BOOK 3

21 MUDRAS FOR AWAKENING CHAKRAS

TABLE OF CONTENTS

Chapter 1. Chakras: How and Why to Awaken Your Chakra 81

Chapter 2. Preparations: Physically, Mentally and Spiritually for a Resurrection Through Awakening Your Chakras........................ 90

Chapter 3. Awakening Your Chakra: Mudras I... 93

Chapter 4. Mudras II............................... 98

Chapter 5. Mudras III............................ 104

Chapter 6. Mudras IV: 110

Chapter 7. Advantages and Disadvantages of Mudras 113

Chapter 8. Keeping Your Chakra Awakened: Tips, Guidelines and Yoga................................. 115

Chapter 9. Conclusion.......................... 117

About The Author 118

Can I Ask A Favour? 118

CHAPTER 1

CHAKRAS: HOW AND WHY TO AWAKEN YOUR CHAKRA

Like the hypotheses, theories, facts and myths of the progressive era denotes, we do not clearly comprehend the semantics of possessing this flawlessly symbiotic life. The mind, though well-known, is never used to the fullest. Simultaneously, the body has the same problem.

Now that we know plenty about amalgamating both, we still are unaware what the fullest is. Chakras, as commonly explained, are the points of focus of the body to trigger, undo, heal and cure directly, and it lies within ourselves. Simply put, if you say that your chiropractor is a darling one, yes! You see 'em! They are the demigods for today's suffering bodies of bones, plastic, paint and flesh. Chiropractors, who are truly talented, can be your ultimate saviors for all halts in life, in all ways!

Chakras are focal points that result in the cause and effect of all organ movement under its territory. Energizing or awakening the chakra results in cleaning up the energy flow as well as moisturizing and brightening its roots. When immersed in the inherent power of mudras and your mind, the body enters a flawlessly abundant flow of energy. There are many mantras to help the situation as well. The effect is emphasized by these chants from the ancient Indian language: Sanskrit. These focal points, as described by the scriptures, do many good when you register them in the bottom of your subconscious.

They are:

1. Root/ Base:

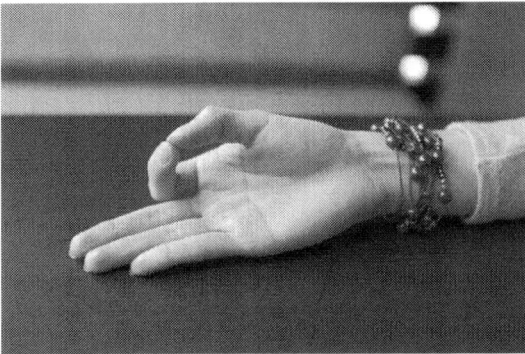

Direction:

    a. Touch the tip of your Index finger with the thumb, deliberately.

    b. Meditate for 12 breaths.

    c. Concentrate on your flow of breath, in and out.

    d. Observe it closely.

    e. Chant the mantra of LAM as much as you can, unhurriedly through the breath.

    f. Focus on the patch of private space in between the anus and the genitalia.

g. The focus should gradually move onto one's own connection to Earth, its gravity and existence. The mudra is geo-targeted.

h. Additionally, any favorite activity that ignites the chakra is worthy to activate higher concentration.

i. Or, stand, relax, widen shoulders, bend your knees, push your pelvis forward, balance yourself with even weight-distribution on soles and sink down. Stay in the same position for 10-15 minutes.

j. Another method of grounding for Root or Base focus is to contract the muscle patch between the anus and the genitalia. Inhale, contract, exhale and relax! Continue for a few minutes. Do anytime.

2. Sacral (Ovaries/ Prostate):

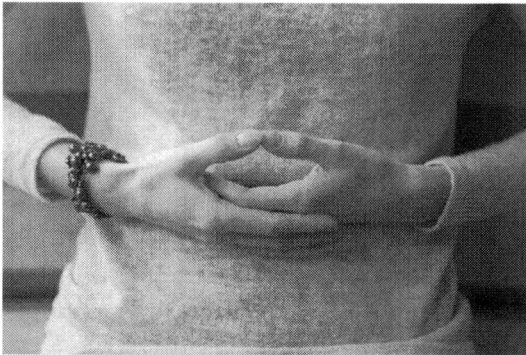

Primarily known as the layer of emotional skeleton, the sacral layer is quintessentially a mudra to focus the energy in the lower back or sacral bone.

a. Sit in a comfortable position.
b. Put both hands in your lap.
c. Keep hands on each other with palms up.
d. Keep your left hand underneath the right.

e. Touch the tip of your fingertips gently onto the immediate skin.
f. During this, chant the mantra VAM.
g. This can help in curing uneven pains and infertility.
h. Another mental advantage of this mudra is healing the creativity block.

3. Solar/ Navel

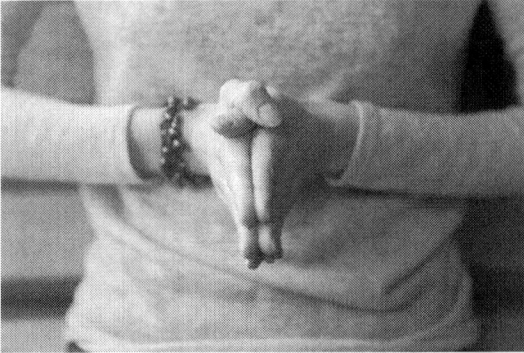

Famed and titled as the intellectual diaphragm, the solar plexus helps in healing many mood swings, intellectual curiosities, enthusiasms, low self-confidence as well as indigestion.

a. Sit down comfortably.
b. Put both your hands in front of your stomach.
c. Cup them horizontal straight.
d. Join your hands firmly by the tips.
e. Cross just the thumbs
f. Straighten the finger and hold it with strong might.
g. The focus is currently on the spine, or precisely put, onto the navel area of our body.
h. The mantra to be chanted during this meditative juncture is RAM.

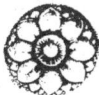

BANYEN
books & sound

Instructive & Artful
Resources for Being,
Loving & Waking Up

Healing Arts,
Spiritual Traditions,
Metaphysics & Meditation,
Yoga & Earth Wisdom,
Poetry & Inspiration

❖

Books, Music, Audios, Videos,
Altar Crafts, Yoga & Healing Tools,
Candles, Incenses & Crystals,
Gifts of Beauty & Heart

❖

3608 West 4th Ave. (at Dunbar)
Vancouver, BC V6R 1P1 Canada
Books: 604-732-7912
Music, Gifts, Events: 604-737-8858
Mail Order: 800-663-8442

banyen.com

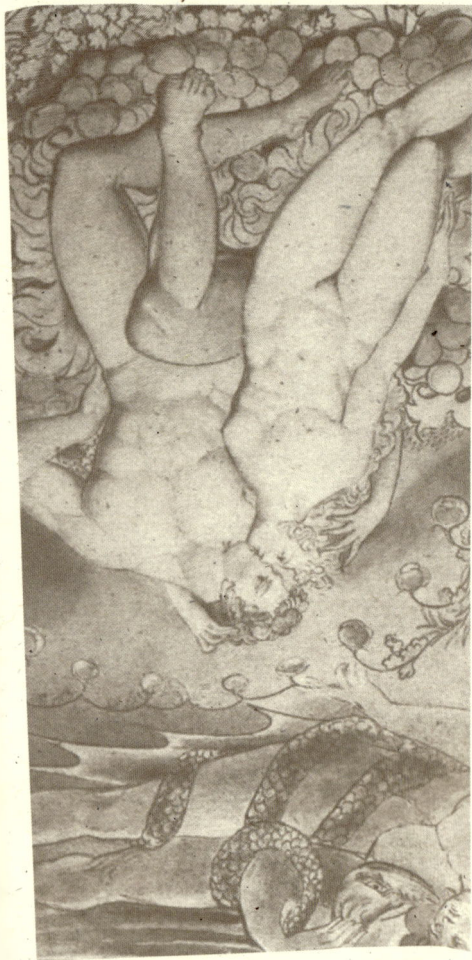

4. Anahata/ Heart/ Cardiac

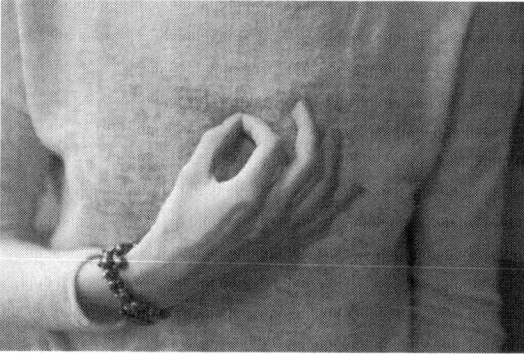

Named as the layer for understanding, empathizing and loving, this mudra focuses on the central force of heart. The main virtues that adorn the mudra are humility, compassion, love and harmony. The chakra also catalyses unbound physical love.

a. Cross your legs and sit.
b. Touch the thumb tip with your index finger of the same hand.
c. Keep this straight ahead of your breast bone.
d. Keep your left hand on your knees.
e. Focus the energy of the chakra to your spine.
f. All through, chant the mantra YAM.

5. Throat/ Vishuddhi

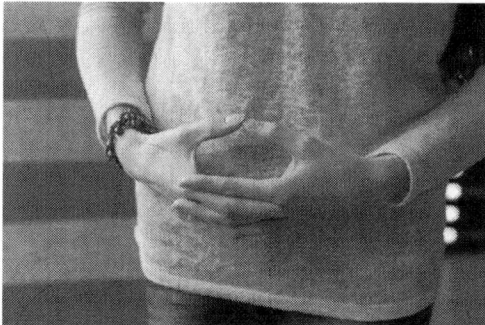

Located in the area between the sternum and chin, Vishuddhi mudra is an embodiment of one's knowledge and its bang. This chakra enhances one's own power of communication and truth through sensible speech.

> a. Inside your hands, cross your fingers, except your thumbs.
> b. Make the thumbs join the tips outside the ball of fingers.
> c. Pull the structure slightly up.
> d. Primary focus while doing this mudra should be on your throat.
> e. The mantra to be hymned is HAM.
> f. Mudra helps one articulate one's feelings without halts or curbs.

6. Third Eye/ Brow/ Ajna

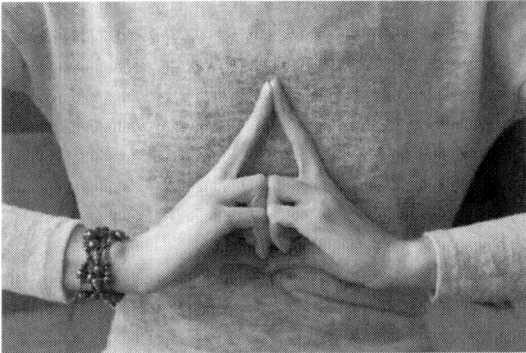

Located right above one's eyes, Ajna chakra is the all-seeing eye of the soul or Third Eye. This energy is termed as a celestial layer as one's innate perception's during this act is beyond the parameters of the physical reality as we see it!

> a. Hold both your hands under your bust.
> b. Join the tip of both your middle fingers by keeping them erect.

c. Bend the rest of your fingers and join at their middle phalanx.

d. The thumbs remain only to join each other by pointing down.

e. The primary focus is on the space above the eyebrows, straight up.

f. During the mudra, chant the mantra OM/ AUM.

g. The mudra focuses on awakening the spiritual insight, enlightenment and lucid reality.

h. The chakra helps in providing poor intuitive abilities and depression.

7. Crown /Temples/ Sahasrara Chakra

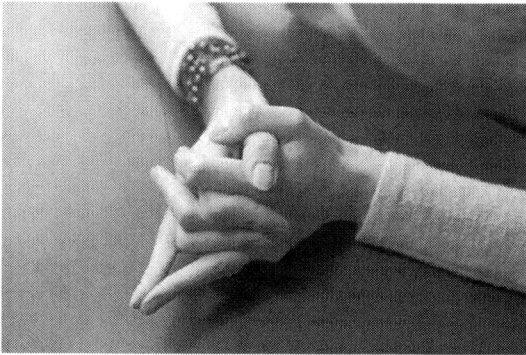

Popularly known as the mastermind of all of life's possibilities and knowledge as well as the soul's own experiences throughout the endless rocking time called lifespan, the causal layer is focused on connecting to "the God" or to "the Creator."

a. Ranges 5 feet away from the body.

b. Always assert strong root chakra before awakening the Sahasrara chakra.

c. Pull your hands in front of your tummy.

d. Point your ring fingers horizontally straight.

e. Touch the tips slightly.

f. Cross the rest of your fingers around each other. (Note: Not the fingertips.)
g. Place the thumb tight and firm underneath the aforementioned.
h. The energy focus is on top of your temples.
i. Chant the mantra NG during the meditation.

Why awaken your chakras?

When the chakras are realized, pampered awake from slumber and charged, your body undergoes an almost docile form of renewal, rejuvenation and reawakening. The fact that this is the lifestyle guaranteed for the transhumant or the enlightened era, suffices that one should care and nourish the flow of energy or the Energy Cogwheels.

Grease 'em up! Clean them with the magic and heat in your fingertips and kick it start!

The how of this question is the certain difficulty, as we see lucidly. Chakra enhances one's consciousness, in and ahead of time. It is interwoven into the fabric of destiny, ability and exploration that dimensions are just a passing feast of the soul!
This proves the worth of being one with the entire infinity so that your soul rises to the level of a spirit that is healthy, awakened and powerfully independent!

A small chakra chart should provide a deeper insight of the advantages of charging up your chakras.

Title	Location	Sense Organ	Reactive Organ	Colour	Air	Syllable
1. Muladhara	Spine-Base	Smell	Cleansing with removal	Red/ Earth	Apana	LAM
2. Sacral	Below abdomen	Taste	Procreation	Orange/ Water	Vyana	VAM
3. Solar	Above Abdomen	Sight	Movement	Yellow/ Fire	Samana	RAM
4. Anahata	Heart	Tactility/ Feeling	Holding/ Grasping/ Comprehension	Green/ Air	Udanu	YAM
5. Vishuddhi	Throat	Audibility	Speech	Blue/ Ether		HAM
6. Ajna	Eyes	Mental	Mind	Indigo		AUM/ OM
8. Sahasrara	Temples	Consciousness	Consciousness/ Subconsciousness	Violet		Silence

All of us have innately blocked chakras in each of us. The way to process your ailment out is through identifying the source of the energy rising, initially. The perfection lies in determining the precise wheels with agony to a sacred land of rejuvenated purity and life!

The chapters ahead provide you with all the knowledge you'll need to become a Master Chakra Awakener through 25 mudras.

CHAPTER 2

PREPARATIONS: PHYSICALLY, MENTALLY AND SPIRITUALLY FOR A RESURRECTION THROUGH AWAKENING YOUR CHAKRAS

Determining the source of cause

Sl No:	Effect	Chakra
a)	Disconnected concentration, difficulty in relaxing/ meditating	Crown
b)	Imbalanced mood swings and heavy headaches, depression	Third Eye
c)	Poor expression skills, detached mind and heart	Throat
d)	High B.P., fear of intimacy and null empathy	Heart
e)	Willpower failure and low self-esteem and confidence, indigestion and low blood sugar	Solar
f)	Lower creativity, low sexual urges, infertility and unbearable periods	Sacral
g)	Unsafe and claustrophobic, fatigue and constipation	Root

Mantras

One of the oldest Indian ways to meditate started with chants. Chants eventually were interwoven into the popular culture of communication as well. As opposed to the fact how sacred and spiritually growing it is to talk, our own individual rants, sirens, abuses and screams are an explicit example of the similar growing. The right mantras focus and relax one's state and can enhance one's own to rectify health and healing.

This very simple technique merely requires ten minutes on a repeated basis. The technique relies on this repetition of mantras that can kick start a meditation instantly in you to focus and see. The word, often a monosyllabic word, is chanted for hours while letting the energy and thoughts flow freely and regardless of the all! This makes the effect primarily on two major levels. Firstly, chakras in and around your mouth cavity can trigger a meditational phase from the positioning of the mouth into the face and tongue. Awakening these is easy as they simply open up after thorough and direct focus through the energy rays.

Make sure you know the comfort and apt pronunciation of the mantra you are chanting. Exemplifying, 'a' is 'ah' and 'o' is 'oh'!

Root	LAM
Sacral	VAM
Solar	RAM
Heart	HAM
Throat	Aum/ OM
Third-eye	NG
Crown	Silence

Mudras:

The second and the foremost preparation we need to heal and to awaken your chakras is the knowledge of mudras. Just as the body is connected well into the Energy Cogwheels, our palms, hand, soles and toes are also connected to control various distances over simple tricks and trips. These mudra chakras directly energize the flow through your body and mind through sufficient throttle and thrust!

91

Take care to practice and learn to hold a single mudra for at least 5 minutes as a stretch.

Poses:

In order to attain a clear and direct flow of energy in your body, you also need to be accumulating all your voluntary control over to the energy focus gradually. All poses and mudras are awakened if performed in a meditative air. Though there are blocks that are too sturdy for the mind to break alone, rejoice in the power of your body and of its health!

Root	Mountain/ Warrior/ Bridge
Sacral	Twist/ Triangle/ Cobra
Solar	Bow/ Full Boat/ Crocodile
Heart	Fish/ Cobra/ Camel
Throat	Upward Plank/ Fish/ Plough
Third Eye	Easy Seat/ Forward Bend / Child's
Crown	Lotus/ Corpse

Color Code:

This code is the result of many great findings that advocate that in order to build up a healthy body that is detoxified, radiant and positive, one must be very much aware of all sides of one's diet and surrender. Below, each color denominates the color of vegetables one must eat, to heat up the designative chakra. Enrich your body with all preparations to open both your mind and body into commonness sans all the weights ever coined by any vocabulary of the world!

Red	Apples, Beets and Pomegranates
Orange	Nuts, Seeds, Oranges and Carrots
Yellow	Lentils (Yellow), Corn and Yellow Sweet Pepper
Green	Leafy Veggies, Kale and Broccoli
Blue	Kelp and Blueberries
Deep Blue	Purple Grapes, Blackberries and Purple Potatoes
Purple	Eggplant and Plum

CHAPTER 3

AWAKENING YOUR CHAKRA: MUDRAS I

As much as the first chapter has instilled the knowledge about chakras in your head, now you need to concentrate on the aspect of mudras.

Some of the mudras to start you off are:

Mudra #1
Dhyana mudra

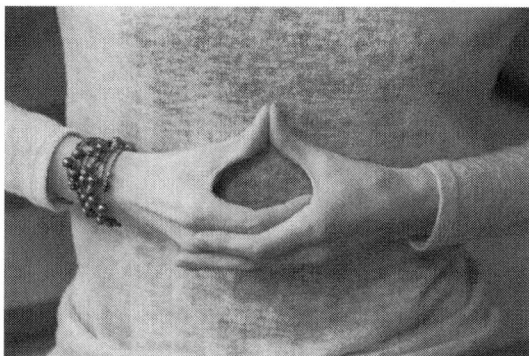

Start concentrating on awakening any chakra, preferably the first or the last.

a. Sit comfortably with both knees positioned horizontally outward and your soles on the opposites, intertwined with the other.
b. Keep your left hand in an open palm with the wrist facing toward the left.
c. Keep your right hand on top on the left hand.
d. Repeat after a session with left hand on top.
e. Keep your thumbs raised and pressed against but together.
f. Be erect and keep your spine stretched.

Mudra #2
Abhaya mudra:

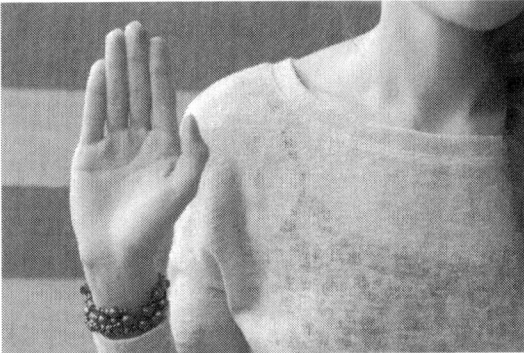

The next step is to "grant absence to your fear," that is, the Abhaya Mudra. It is performed in teaching definite and higher ends of meditation.

a. Sit comfortably.
b. Focus on your mind chakra.
c. Flow without a fear of death and rebirth.
d. Keep your left hand rested on your thighs or its ends.
e. Keep your right hand raised up to your shoulder.
f. Face your palm towards the outside.

Mudra #3
Vyakarana Mudra

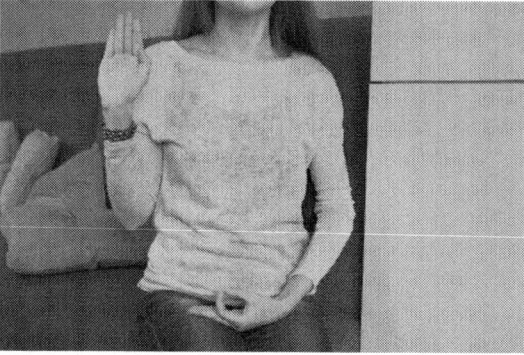

This is the ultimate mudra of the psychic for the power of universal prediction. This mudra is all about the phase of enlightenment and its focus and is the combined energy of two mudras.

    a. Firstly, perform Abhaya Mudra with your right hand.

    b. Now perform Orna or Wool Mudra with your left hand (grasp the hems of your fabric/ garment or loose cloak).

Mudra #4
Dharmachakra Mudra

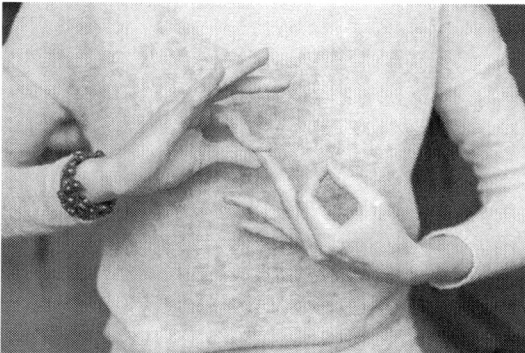

An unusual and unrecorded combination of chakra, Dharmachakra refines to a mode of enlightenment that is almost instant.

1. Hold your right hand in front of your chest, almost touching it.
2. Be straight in your comfortable posture.
3. Now bring your left-hand fingers straight and erect to be held by the right hand in the posture.
4. Keep your thumbs protruding out.
5. All through, continue focusing and charging your chakra to awaken yourself.

Mudra #5
Anjalimudra

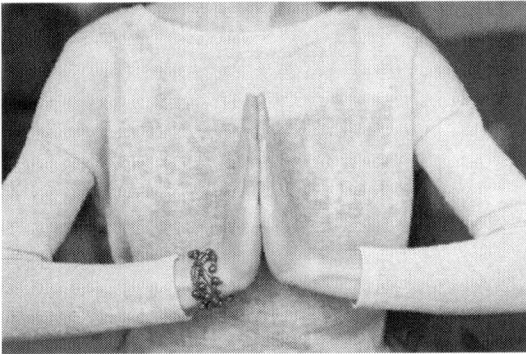

One of the most sacred mudras, this is the most prominent mudra in India, as a symbol for Namaskar or wishing. Used prominently to greet or to respect anyone and everyone, the gesture is a prominent mudra to awaken and charge your chakra.

1. Clap both your hands straight in front of your chest.
2. Sit in a comfortable position.
3. Focus on your chakra and charge it with your energy that circles the self.

Mudra #6
Varada Mudra

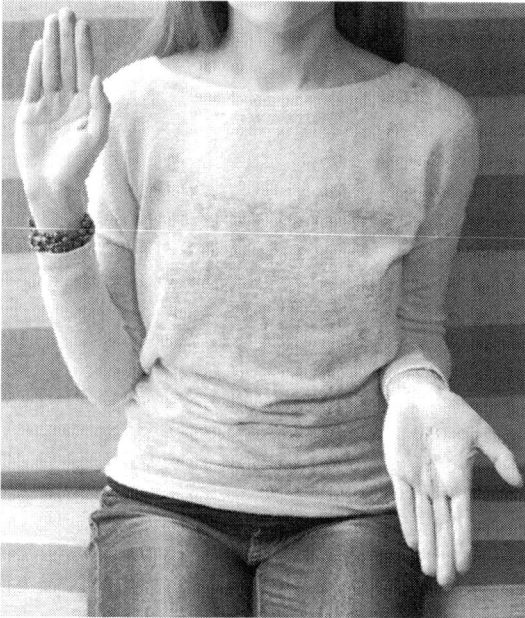

The gesture to start, begin or permit, Varada Mudra is an emphatic flow of positivity. Stand in a comfortable position and focus on your chakra to begin.

1. Hold both your hands parallel to your standing body.
2. Now hold the wrists to the left and right, away from the body, respectively.
3. The idea is to hold a gesture equivalent to bestowal.
4. Arch your palm and fingers to add to the charge and focus of your chakra.

CHAPTER 4

MUDRAS II

As per the Buddhist scriptures, a mudra is a seal or stamping ring that is impressed, usually, upon a body.

Mudra #7
Pran

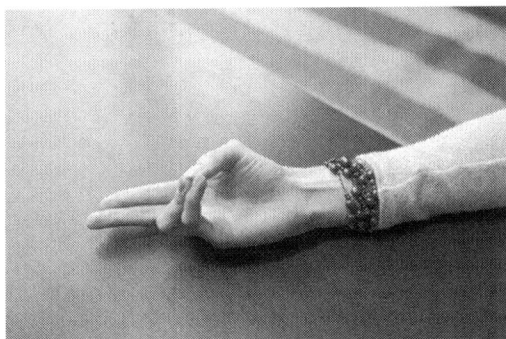

Generally known as the mudra of life.

    a. Place the tips of your little finger, ring finger and thumb together.
    b. Keep the index finger pointing straight out.
    c. Do this for half an hour with changing central positions and focus.

d. This mudra is performed to instigate vision, attentiveness and fatigue.
e. Create a focus by believing that you yourself is a tree.
f. Inhale and exhale by charging in and out of your chakra.

Mudra #8
Linga

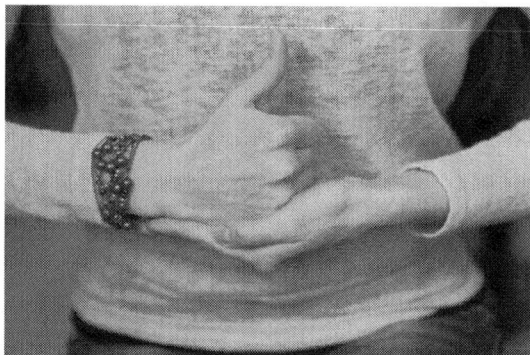

Generally known as the upright mudra.

a. Stand up.
b. Spread your legs slightly.
c. Bend your knees slightly.
d. Inhale with keeping your head to the right.
e. Exhale with turning your head to the left.
f. Place both palms in front of you.
g. Clasp your fingers against each other.
h. Start by keeping one of your thumbs to the right, protruding out.
i. Encircle this particular outward finger with the index and thumb finger of your other hand.
j. Do the same and charge your chakra for 20 minutes as many times a day as you wish.
k. This is a good mudra to boost your chakra for immunity.

Mudra #9
Apan

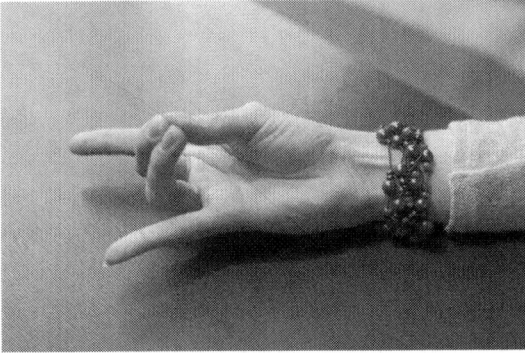

Generally titled as the mudra of energy, Apan is easy to do.

a. On each hand, hold the tips of your ring finger, middle finger and thumb together.
b. Place them outwards with respect to your body.
c. Extend the rest of your fingers.
d. Do at least 30 minutes each per day thrice.
e. This mudra instigates the removal of all your anti or negative energy to nourish, strengthen and nurture your awakened chakra.
f. The precise organs healed during this are the galls and bladder. It also works to balance your harmony with the nature and reality around you.

Mudra #10
Shankh

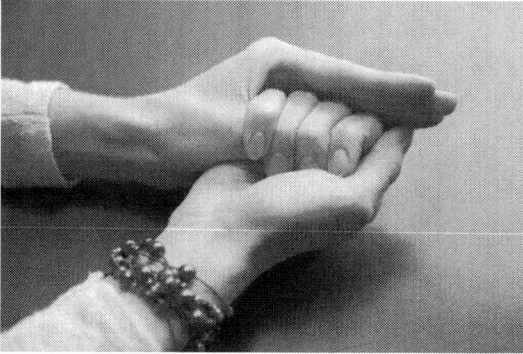

Generally titled as the mudra of shell, Shankh
represents opening.

a. Encircle the four fingers of your right hand
with the thumb protruding out.
b. Place the palm of your left hand against the
fist of your right and touch the tip of your
right-hand thumb with the left-hand little
finger.
c. Practice this mudra alongside a perpetual
chanting of the mantra "OM."
d. This mudra opens up the dirt and misfortune
of our physical, spiritual, emotional and
perspective-based realities.

Mudra #11
Surabhi

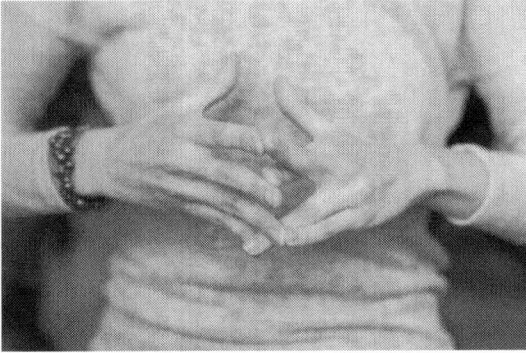

Generally termed as the cow mudra, this awakens and heals the energy related to movement. ,

- a. Tip of your little finger on the left hand touches the ring finger on the right hand.
- b. Tip of your little finger on the right hand touches the ring finger on the left hand.
- c. Now touch the tip of your middle finger of both hands to touch the index fingertips of the other.
- d. Keep your thumbs open and straight.
- e. Do at least ten times per day thrice.
- f. For all sorts of physical, mental and emotional aches, one should practice this mudra.

Mudra #12
Vayu

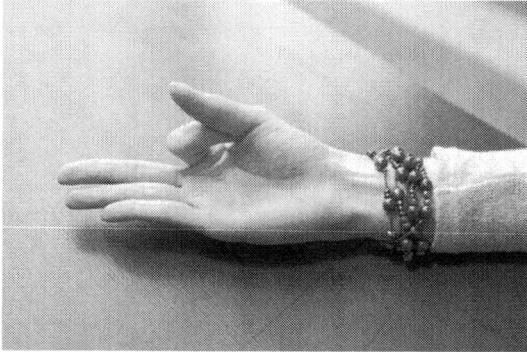

Generally titled as the wind mudra, Vayu can clean and heal a lot of the chronic complaint a person has about his personal body, health and mind.

    a. With the tip of your index finger, bend to touch the ball of your thumb inside the palm.
    b. Now fold your thumbs over the index and tighten slightly.
    c. Straighten out your remaining fingers in a relaxed position.
    d. Do this for at least 15 minutes per day thrice.
    e. This mudra is known to heal zillions of the wind and respiratory illnesses as well as ventilating one's mind.
    f. This also cleans up the waste that has accumulated due to too much wind on previous accounts.

CHAPTER 5

MUDRAS III

Mudras are elaborate in the Buddhist world and are used in a position to concentrate with the interwoven fingers and bodily positions to make sense and to possess a magical efficacy.

Mudra #13
Shunya

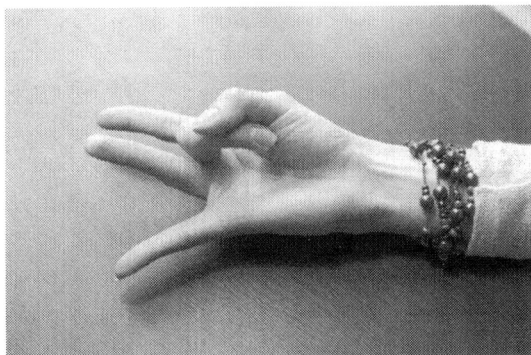

Generally called the heaven mudra, Shunya is the core of the treatment methods to charge up your chakra. It clears your chakras for the strength of your ears and its hearing disorders.

a. Bend both your middle fingers and press them onto the ball of your thumbs.
b. Now fold your thumb to seal this, gently.
c. Keep your other fingers all extended.
d. Do this with each hand separately for half an hour thrice.
e. This mudra opens up the ultimate gateway (middle finger) to heaven.
f. Practice regularly and thoroughly.

Mudra #14
Prithvi

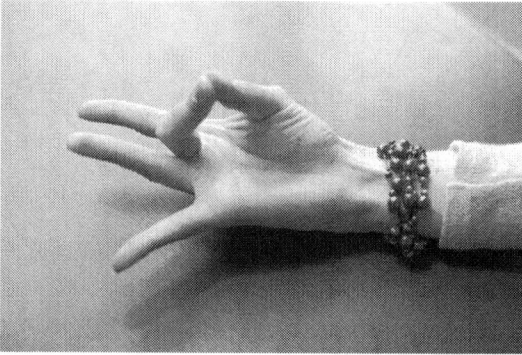

Generally called the mudra of Earth, Prithvi has to do much with your root chakra. Prithvi ignites your base passion, energy and power to charge your chakras brighter.

a. Hold the tips of your ring finger and thumb on top of one another.
b. Apply a light pressure.
c. Extend the remaining fingers.
d. Practice this with each of your hands for 20 minutes, 2-3 times daily.
e. This mudra provides roots of stability and charge for your chakra to remain lit.

Mudra #15
Varuna

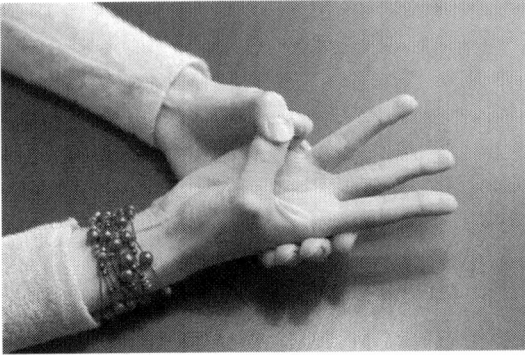

Generally called the mudra of water, this mudra is exclusive during the winter times when there is too much mucus in our body and tummy. This congestion is resolved through charging your chakra around the nasal cavities and lungs.

a. Fold the little finger of your right hand
b. Now stretch it to touch the tip of your left-hand thumb ball.
c. Now pull the thumb of your left hand and bend it around the other hand, in order to keep it slightly pressured on the bended little finger.
d. Practice for 10 minutes, 5 times daily.
e. This mudra helps in removing all stimulations, accumulations and congestions in the body and mind.

Mudra #16
Bhudi

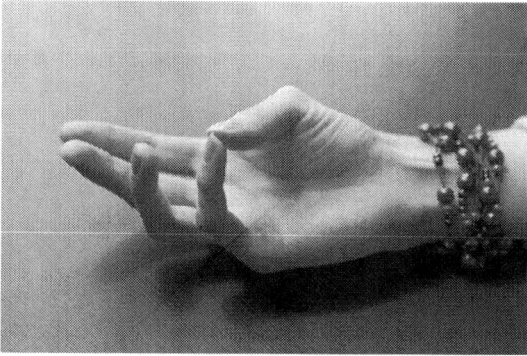

Generally titled as the fluid mudra, this helps to create equilibrium throughout the body with respect to its fluids.

a. Touch your thumb tip and little finger together, gently.
b. Straighten your other fingers in the most relaxed of ways.
c. Continue to do this with each of your hands for up to 15 minutes thrice daily.
d. This mudra is used to heal dryness and heal the sense of taste.

Mudra #17
Apan Vayu

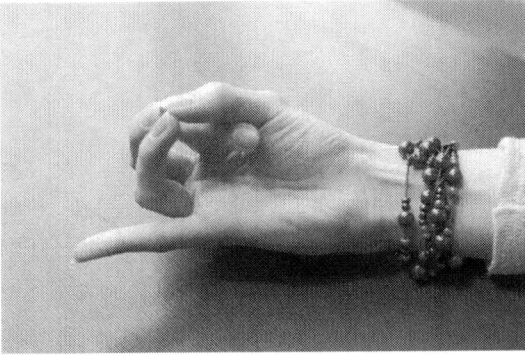

Generally titled as the lifesaver mudra, this is also the most primitive first aid. The finger positions are held in such a way that it regulates the strengthening for your heart. For a cardiac arrest, you have little or null time.

a. Fold your index finger to touch the ball of your palm.
b. Touch your middle finger's tip and the tip of your ring finger to touch the thumb tip.
c. Now, extend your little fingers.
d. Continue the exercise twice with each finger by spending 20 minutes each.
e. This mudra is used to heal oneself, and listening to music does halve the effect.

Mudra #18
Suchi

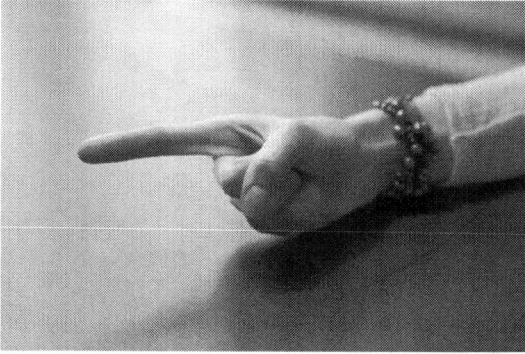

Generally used for bowel-related problems and aches in your tummy, Suchi mudra is used to resolve constipation-related issues.

a. Clench both your fists tightly.
b. Hold them straight in front of your chest.
c. Inhale with your index finger of the right hand pointed outward.
d. Stretch your arms as well.
e. Stretch to the right with your left arm.
f. Hold this precise tension for 6 long breaths and return to the fundamental position.
g. When it comes to internal cleaning, Suchi mudra has the maximum effect.

CHAPTER 6

MUDRAS IV:

In Chinese cultures, Mudras are known as the personal distinguishing signature or mark that one implies.

Mudra #19
Matangi

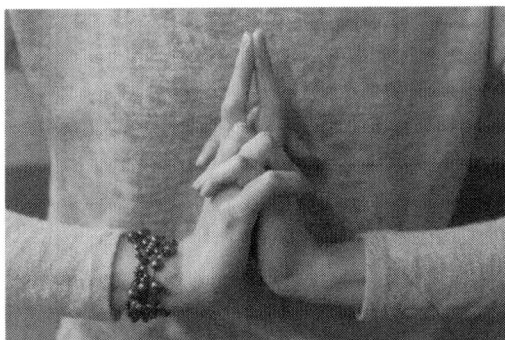

Generally titled the god of our inner harmony and leadership, Matangi mudra is used to enhance and enrich respiration. This mudra is used to catalyze the wood element to trigger a new starting. The theory holds to excite and activate the inner energy to empty all confusions.

a. Fold both your hands and hold it in front of your tummy.
b. Point both of your middle fingers outside.
c. Keep your hands against each other all the while.
d. Focus your chakra or charge it up by thinking about it.
e. This mudra primarily focuses one's own inner energies.

Mudra #20
Mahasirs

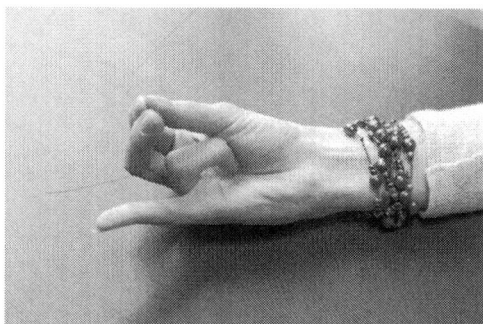

Generally titled as the large head mudra for curing persistent headaches once and for all. The tension in your head, eyes or other sense organs can be easily resolved through chakra charging through mudras.

a. Touch the thumb tip, middle finger and index finger against each other.
b. Fold your ring finger into the fold of your thumb.
c. Keep your little finger straightened out and protruded.
d. Conduct this exercise with each of your hands at a stretch of about 20 minutes thrice every day.
e. This mudra is used to relieve and balance the energy in you.

111

Mudra #21
Hakini

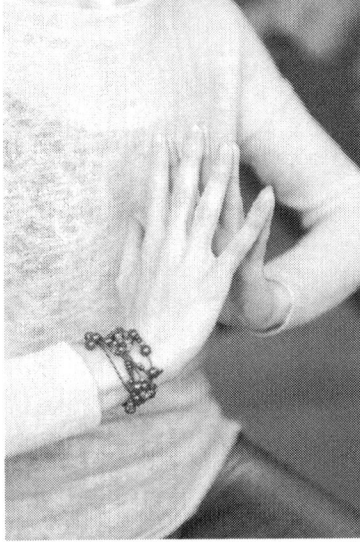

Generally named as the god of forehead, this is one of the most important mudras to awaken your chakras. This mudra also helps in simultaneously charging your chakra.

a. Sit comfortably.
b. Place all the tips of your fingers against each other.
c. Now concentrate on your chakra and charge it up!
d. This mudra is used to enhance memory, increase concentration and alertness.
e. While doing the mudra, that is, while inhaling, place your tongue tip on your gums.
f. While exhaling, let the tongue down.
g. This also stimulates extreme cooperation between the right and left hemispheres of the brain.

CHAPTER 7

ADVANTAGES AND DISADVANTAGES OF MUDRAS

Mudras are just as any other physical medicine—when taken with care and special diet, they render amazing healing, unlike the mixed failed result when combined with alcohol and a disordered lifestyle. Although the advantages weigh out the disadvantages, it is necessary to understand that all the aspects of mindfulness can render both advantages and disadvantages.

There are umpteen advantages of mudras in all of our day-to-day lives. We can use mudras to heal our physical ailments, mental halts and emotional blocks. Mudras are used to clear out the boulders in the paths of our waking hours and dreams. Mudras can be used to reduce considerable weight, relax, reduce stress and eliminate fears as well as physical diseases. From unlocking fluid-filled cavities, to clearing the blocks that have blocked the smooth flow of energy inside us, mudras help in healing almost all of your problems. Practicing these mudras three-four times for about 20 minutes each day will clear you out of all your aches and ailments.

However, the focus is that not all these awakened chakra, the body and the spirit will do well when you're abiding to the poor lifestyle options that do more damage than good. These are not the lone disadvantages of mudras, but these can render long-lasting and deep damages if you combine them with an undisciplined and uneven routine around the activity of relaxation, mediation and chakra awakening.

When mudras are regularly practiced with a fixed duration and timing, the regularity strikes a discipline in the person that is uplifting, health and hygiene wise. Often times, the stress in our heads and bodies drives us toxic and confused to heap up more diseases. One should opt out for relaxation techniques of yoga and other mudra mode of meditation.

CHAPTER 8

KEEPING YOUR CHAKRA AWAKENED: TIPS, GUIDELINES AND YOGA

In order to keep the charged and awakened chakra perpetually active, one must try to follow many tips and guidelines apart from following your own concentration method of focusing.

Some symbols to know beforehand are the lock symbol, which means to hold a secret. The hand itself signifies many Hindu gods. It also signifies many other states of minds such as anger, regret, joyfulness and serenity. To make your body as well as mind flexible to battle and resolve all tensions, one must practice chakra charging and awakening regularly and in a healthy way. Just like the locked fingers, thumb and its pressure, determine the focus of the cosmic energy, through practice and regular energy flow, and then your health and radiance will start strengthening.

Another important aspect one should note by this stage of practice is the right way of breathing. This aspect of re-birthing breathing depends on a rapid and a shallow breath that involves inhaling strongly while exhalation is conducted in a very relaxed way. After every attempt of this, do thrice-directed breaths. Directed breaths are carried out through inhalation and exhalation in a relaxed and natural way with closed eyes. While respiration is directed, one should imagine the pattern of airflow inside and outside his or her body.

1. All mudras can be performed when lying down, sitting, standing or leaning;
2. Mudras should be performed to heal as its focus in its due course.
3. When sitting and performing a mudra, sit upright with an erect spine.
4. Let your hands relax on your thighs.
5. Pull your chin a little back; keep your neck long and erect.

Some tips for the chakras are the focal points when charging your chakra:

a. Root: Spine Base
b. Sacral: Navel
c. Solar: Stomach
d. Heart: Lungs and Heart
e. Throat: Throat and Mouth
f. Third Eye: Eyebrows
g. Crown: Temples

CHAPTER 9

CONCLUSION

Thank you for downloading this book.

I wish you all the good luck, peace and mind power to excel and find great fortune in oneself through awakened and charged chakras through mudras to heal and restore the health of your body, soul and mind. Make sure your regularity, discipline and flow of energy are never put to any halts from now on!

Good Luck!

About The Author

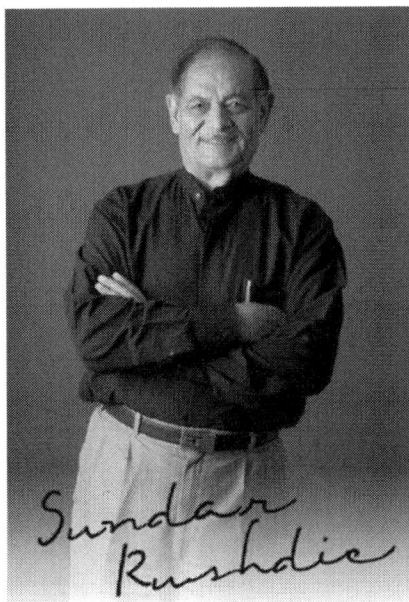

Sundar Rushdie is an author, healer and researcher of ancient Indian practices.

During the long years of research, he got a wealth of experience and knowledge in such practices as yoga, mudras and ayurveda.

In his spare time between research, practice and writing books, he enjoys spending time with his family—three children and five grandchildren.

CAN I ASK A FAVOUR?

If you enjoyed this book, found it useful or otherwise then I'd really appreciate it if you would post a short review on Amazon. I do read all the reviews personally so that I can continually write what people are wanting.

Thanks for your support!

Made in the USA
San Bernardino, CA
15 September 2016